The Jossey-Bass Health Series brings together the most current information and ideas in health care from the leaders in the field. Titles from the Jossey-Bass Health Series include these essential health care resources:

Creating Excellence in Crisis Care: A Guide to Effective Training and Program Designs
Lee Ann Hoff, Kazimiera Adamowski

Curing Health Care: New Strategies for Quality Improvement
Donald M. Berwick, A. Blanton Godfrey, Jane Roessner

Profiting from Quality: Outcomes Strategies for Medical Practice
Steven F. Isenberg, Richard E. Gliklich, Editors

Raising Standards in American Health Care: Best People, Best Practices, Best Results
V. Clayton Sherman

Restructuring Health Care: The Patient-Focused Paradigm
J. Philip Lathrop, Booz*Allen Health Care, Inc.

Status One: Breakthroughs in High Risk Population Health Management
Samuel Forman, Matthew Kelliher

The Juran Prescription: Clinical Quality Management
Kathleen Jennison Goonan

Through the Patient's Eyes: Understanding and Promoting Patient-Centered Care
Margaret Gerteis, Susan Edgman-Levitan, Jennifer Daley, Thomas L. Delbanco, Editors

Total Customer Satisfaction: A Comprehensive Approach for Health Care Providers
Stephanie G. Sherman, V. Clayton Sherman

Total Quality in Healthcare: From Theory to Practice
Ellen J. Gaucher, Richard J. Coffey

CULTURAL
COMPETENCE
IN HEALTH CARE

A PRACTICE GUIDE

CULTURAL

COMPETENCE

IN HEALTH CARE

A PRACTICE GUIDE

Editors

Anne Rundle

Maria Carvalho and Mary Robinson

Children's Hospital, Boston

An earlier version of this book was previously published in
hard binder format under the title *Honoring Patient Preferences*

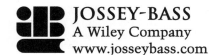

JOSSEY-BASS
A Wiley Company
www.josseybass.com

Published by

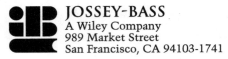

JOSSEY-BASS
A Wiley Company
989 Market Street
San Francisco, CA 94103-1741

www.josseybass.com

Jossey-Bass books and products are available through most bookstores. To contact Jossey-Bass directly, call (888) 378-2537, fax to (800) 605-2665, or visit our website at www.josseybass.com.

Substantial discounts on bulk quantities of Jossey-Bass books are available to corporations, professional associations, and other organizations. For details and discount information, contact the special sales department at Jossey-Bass.

We at Jossey-Bass strive to use the most environmentally sensitive paper stocks available to us. Our publications are printed on acid-free recycled stock whenever possible, and our paper always meets or exceeds minimum GPO and EPA requirements.

Library of Congress Cataloging-in-Publication Data

Honoring Patient Preferences: a guide to complying with multicultural patient requirements / Anne Knights Rundle, Maria Carvalho, Mary Robinson, editors; Children's Hospital, Boston.—1st ed.

    p.   cm.
Includes bibliographical references (p.) and index.
ISBN 0-7879-4650-8 (binder set, original version)
ISBN 0-7879-6221-X (paperback version)
   1. Transcultural medical care—Handbooks, manuals, etc. I. Rundle, Anne Knights, 1965–   II. Carvalho, Maria, 1952–   III. Robinson, Mary, 1951–
RA418.5.T73 H65 1999
362.1—dc21

                                             99-06601
                                               CIP

FIRST EDITION
PB Printing   10 9 8 7 6 5 4 3 2 1

Table of Contents

Preface

AT CHILDREN'S HOSPITAL in Boston, providers see families from many different cultures and religions each day. In order to assist staff members in caring for this diverse patient population, a multidisciplinary committee consisiting of staff whose backgrounds, experience, and careers had evolved from diverse cultural and spiritual backgrounds and from working with diverse patient groups, developed a special guide. The model was introduced in hospital units at staff rounds, using real-life case stories that produced thoughtful problem-solving discussions.

The guide was selected for an award for innovation from The Healthcare Assembly in 1998, where many hospital administrators from around the country, particularly those seeing a new influx of immigrants, expressed a need for guidance in meeting the needs of families from diverse cultural or spiritual backgrounds. *Honoring Patient Preferences* is an improvement and expansion on the original guide. It offers basic information on the general characteristics and traditions of several cultural and religious groups, selected to reflect the most common preferences of the cultures most likely to be seen by a large urban hospital.

Health care organizations using this guide may find cultural or spiritual communities not included in the book, such as the Hmong community. If so, they are invited to use the templates provided in Chapter 11 to create their own guidelines for dealing with other groups. To assist health care providers interested in developing a similar curriculum for their respective organizations, a list of resources, such as consultants, interpreter services, and external agencies, is also provided at the end of the book. Tips for meeting the Joint Commission on Accreditation of Healthcare Organizations (JCAHO) requirements are given in Chapter 12.

We would like to thank the following individuals: Judith Mitiguy for her editing expertise; Dr. Arthur Kleinman and Reverend Mary Martha Thiel for their knowledge and support; Andy Pasternack, Dr. Louise Christian, and Dr. L. W. Bombrake for their guidance; and Emily King, Lindy King, and Katie Crouch for their administrative help.

About the Editors

ANNE RUNDLE, R.N., M.S., formerly a coordinator of family service programs at Children's Hospital in Boston, is a nurse and instructor at the Simmons Graduate School of Health Studies in Boston.

MARIA CARVALHO is a licensed independent clinical social worker and head social worker of the Spanish team. She has been on staff at Children's Hospital, Boston, for the past sixteen years, working primarily with Spanish and Portuguese-speaking families.

REVEREND MARY ROBINSON, M.A., M.Div., is the director of the Department of Pastoral Care at Children's Hospital, Boston.

Editors and Consultants

Editors

Senior Editor

Anne Rundle, R.N., M.S., Manager of Specialty Programs, South End Community Health Center, Boston, MA.

Writer/Editors

Maria Carvalho, LICSW, Social Worker, Children's Hospital, Boston, MA.

Rev. Mary Robinson, M.A., M.Div., Director of Pastoral Care, Children's Hospital, Boston, MA.

Eduardo Berinstein, Manager of Interpreter Services, Children's Hospital, Boston, MA.

Helen Clinton, LICSW, Director of Social Work, Children's Hospital, Boston, MA.

Eileen Hession Laband, R.N., M.B.A., Project Manager, Children's Hospital, Boston, MA.

Consultants

Mojisola Akinola, Nursing Student and Executive Director of the Nigerian Youth Organization of Massachusetts. (Chapter 1, Nigeria)

Jacqueline Almestica, Children's Hospital, Boston, MA. (Chapter 2, Central America and Mexico, Dominican Republic; Chapter 7, Puerto Rico)

Zarita Araujo, Winchester, MA. (Chapter 4, Portugal)

Magdalena Barbosa, Children's Hospital, Belmont, MA. (Chapter 6, Brazil)

Bishop Grant Bennett, The Church of Jesus Christ of Latter-day Saints, Belmont, MA, ward. (Chapter 10, Mormon)

4xvi   Editors and Consultants

Barbara Blundell, Volunteer Services, Children's Hospital, Boston, MA. (Chapter 4, Gypsies)

Ana Margarita Cebollero, Ph.D., Children's Hospital, Boston, MA. (Chapter 7, Puerto Rico)

Bishop Timothy W. Chopeles, The Church of Jesus Christ of Latter-day Saints, Lynnfield, MA, ward. (Chapter 10, Mormon)

Janis Cole, Boston Center for Deaf and Hard-of-Hearing Children, Boston, MA. (Chapter 8, Deaf or Hard-of-Hearing)

Terrell Clark, Ph.D., Boston Center for Deaf and Hard-of-Hearing Children, Boston, MA. (Chapter 8, Deaf or Hard-of-Hearing)

Jessica Henderson Daniel, Ph.D., Children's Hospital, Boston, MA. (Chapter 7, African American)

Bartolomeu De Barros, Interpreter Services, Children's Hospital, Boston, MA. (Chapter 1, Cape Verde)

Roland E. Dennis, Hospital Liaison Committee, Jehovah's Witnesses, 32 Lombard Street, Malden, MA. (Chapter 10, Jehovah's Witness)

Joanne Dunn, North American Indian Center, Boston, MA. (Chapter 7, Native American)

Imam Talal Eid, M.Ed., Muslim Chaplain, Children's Hospital, Boston, MA. (Chapter 10, Islam)

Gregory Figaro, Interpreter Services, Children's Hospital, Boston, MA. (Chapter 3, Haiti)

Keiko Fukasawa, Student, Wheelock College, Boston, MA. (Chapter 2, Japan)

Carlotta Gilarde, CSJ, Catholic Chaplain, Children's Hospital, Boston, MA. (Chapter 10, Roman Catholicism)

Suzanne Graca, M.S., CCLS, Child Life Services, Children's Hospital, Boston, MA. (Chapter 2, Japan)

Sandra Helmers, M.D., Children's Hospital, Boston, MA. (Chapter 8, Families with Gay or Lesbian Parents)

John Hudson, Children's Hospital Family Advisory Committee, Boston, MA. (Chapter 7, African American)

Raja Jahan, Ph.D., Boston, MA. (Chapter 2, India)

Gary Jones, Manager, Committee on Publication, the First Church of Christ, Scientist, Boston, MA. (Chapter 10, First Church of Christ, Scientist)

Deanne Kelleher, R.D., Clinical Dietitian Specialist, Children's Hospital, Boston, MA.

Madeline Ko-i Bastis, Zen Priest, Peaceful Dwelling Project, 2 Harborview Drive, East Hampton, NY. (Chapter 10, Buddhism)

Mark Korson, M.D., Children's Hospital, Boston, MA. (Chapter 8, Families with Gay or Lesbian Parents)

Father Nicholas Krommydas, Greek Orthodox Diocese of Boston. (Chapter 10, Eastern Orthodox)

Ambrizeth Lima, Boston Public Schools, Boston, MA. (Chapter 1, Cape Verde)

Leroy Littlebear, Harvard Native American Program, Boston, MA. (Chapter 7, Native American)

Sheela Magge, M.D., Department of Medicine, Children's Hospital, Boston, MA. (Chapter 10, Hinduism)

Fred Mandell, M.D., Department of Medicine, Children's Hospital, Boston, MA (Chapter 4, Gypsies)

Fatima Martins, Cambridge, MA. (Chapter 4, Portugal)

Maurice Melchiono, R.N., M.S., FNP; Pediatric Health Associates, Children's Hospital, Boston, MA. (Chapter 8, Families with Gay or Lesbian Parents)

Richard Minear, Professor of Japanese History, University of Massachusetts, Amherst, MA. (Chapter 2, Japan)

Jacqueline Miranda, LICSW, Department of Social Work, Children's Hospital, Boston, MA. (Chapter 7, Puerto Rico)

Svein Myreng, Dharmacharya, Melfllombolgen 26, N-1157 Oslo, Norway. (Chapter 10, Buddhism)

Tot Nguyen, Department of Interpreter Services, Children's Hospital, Boston, MA. (Chapter 2, Asia)

Mary O'Malley, R.N., staff nurse, Preoperative Clinic, Children's Hospital, Boston, MA.

Sunday O. Oluokun, Student, University of Ibadam, Nigeria. (Chapter 1, Nigeria)

Mark J. Ott, M.D., Massachusetts General Hospital, Boston, MA. (Chapter 10, Church of Jesus Christ of Latter-day Saints)

Father Angelo Pappas, St. Nicholas Greek Orthodox Church, Portsmouth, NH. (Chapter 10, Eastern Orthodox)

Bess Pappas, Department of Volunteers, Children's Hospital, Boston, MA. (Chapter 4, Greece)

Luanne Pelosi, R.N., M.S., P.N.P., Surgical Nurse Practitioner, Children's Hospital, Boston, MA.

Matilde Peña, Department of Social Work, Children's Hospital, Boston, MA. (Chapter 3, Dominican Republic)

Grace Peters, Department of Interpreter Services, Children's Hospital, Boston, MA.

Saly Pin-Riebe, M.S.W., Office of Multicultural Services Refugee Assistance Plan, Massachusetts Department of Mental Health, Boston, MA. (Chaper 2, Cambodia)

Anna Ribeiro Pinto, M.D., Department ofo Medicine, Children's Hospital, Boston, MA. (Chapter 6, Brazil)

Antonio Magalhaes Pinto, Cambridge, MA. (Chapter 4, Portugal)

Rosamaria Cardoso Pinto, Cambridge, MA. (Chapter 4, Portugal)

Steve Quintana III, Priest of Yoruba Religion, Cuban Santero, Boston, MA. (Chapter 10, Santería)

Maria Rivera, Department of Interpreter Services, Children's Hospital, Boston, MA. (Chapter 3, Dominican Republic; Chapter 7, Puerto Rico)

Jennifer Robertson, Narragansett Tribal Nation and Children's Hospital, Boston, MA. (Chapter 7, Native American)

Eva Sanchez, Department of Interpreter Services, Children's Hospital, Boston, MA. (Chapter 3, Dominican Republic; Chapter 7, Puerto Rico)

Betty Singer, LICSW, Department of Social Work, Children's Hospital, Boston, MA. (Chapter 10, Judaism)

Joao Soares, MD, Massachusetts Alliance of Portuguese Speakers, Somerville, MA. (Chapter 1, Cape Verde)

Israel Sokeye, Medical Student, University of Ibadam, Nigeria. (Chapter 1, Nigeria)

Jody Steiner, ASL Interpreter, Children's Hospital, Boston, MA. (Chapter 8, Deaf or Hard-of-Hearing)

Katie Sultan, R.N., Staff Nurse, Emergency Department, Children's Hospital, Boston, MA.

Gunga Tavares, Cultural Attache, Consulate of Cape Verde, Boston, MA. (Chapter 1, Cape Verde)

Rev. Mary Martha Thiel, Department of Pastoral Care, Massachusetts General Hospital, Boston, MA. (Chapter 10, Religions)

Judith Toyama, Director of Graduate Student Recruitment and Retention, University of Massachusetts, Amherst, MA. (Chapter 2, Japan)

Lac Tran, Chief Information Officer, Children's Hospital, Boston, MA. (Chapter 2, Vietnam)

Irina Vatman, Department of Interpreter Services, Children's Hospital, Boston, MA. (Chapter 4, Russia)

Isabel Vazquez, M.S., R.D., Clinical Dietitian Specialist, Children's Hospital, Boston, MA.

Manuel Vilar, Department of Interpreter Services, Children's Hospital, Boston, MA. (Chapter 2, Portugal; Chapter 1, Cape Verde)

Rabbi Jerome Weistrop, D.Min, Jewish Chaplain, Children's Hospital, Boston, MA. (Chapter 10, Judaism)

Sunela Wikramanayake, Wheelock College Student Intern, Children's Hospital, Boston, MA. (Chapter 1, Nigeria)

Peter Wolff, M.D., Department of Medicine, Children's Hospital, Boston, MA. (Chapter 1, Eritrea)

Rev. Elinor Yeo, M.Div., Protestant Chaplain, Children's Hospital, Boston, MA. (Chapter 10, Protestantism)

Introduction

EFFECTIVE HEALTH CARE incorporates the cultural traditions and spiritual concerns of the patient and his or her family. Children's Hospital, Boston, has developed this guide to help health care providers improve relationships with patients and families who represent an increasingly diverse population. The guide offers basic information on the general characteristics and traditions of several cultural and religious groups. It also contains information on resources, such as consultants, interpreter services, and external agencies, and tips for meeting requirements of the Joint Commission on Accreditation of Healthcare Organizations (JCAHO).

Although the guide's objective is to acquaint providers with the traditions of their cultures, the authors urge readers to first consider their own value systems, as the providers' own traditions, values, belief systems, and biases may affect their care of a patient who has different cultural norms. In the United States, many providers are educated in Western traditional medicine, which promotes certain values about health and illness. Usually, biological (or biomedical) information is of primary concern, sometimes to the exclusion of all other aspects. For example, a provider with Western training may not appreciate a family's reliance on a spiritual healer. It is essential to remember that a patient's and his or her family's perception and understanding of the origin and meaning of well-being, illness, and recovery can be major factors in the health care process.

Culture of the Health Care Provider

Many of the providers at Children's Hospital are Caucasian North Americans or "Western." Although they are as diverse as any other ethnic group, there are some similarities in Western culture that set members apart from other cultural groups. For example, communication style among most North Americans tends to be linear, direct, and "to-the-point." In other cultures, such as African, Asian, and Latino, communication may be a more narrative form, and people may get to the point gradually. In Western culture, direct eye contact is a sign of respect and attentiveness, whereas in other cultures it may be considered disrespectful or an affront.

In Western culture, people value time-efficient behavior. Time is "saved," "lost," or "wasted." It is very important to be "on time"; Western thinking is often future-oriented. People plan for the future in many aspects of their lives. Believing that they, not fate, control the environment, they think they can determine the direction of many areas of their lives. In many other cultures, time is present-oriented or past-oriented. Taking time to build personal relationships is much more important than being "on time"; therefore, stopping to talk to a neighbor could be more important than arriving on time for a clinic appointment.

Although preventive medicine is an important aspect of health care in the United States, in many other countries it is simply not practiced. For example, a Central American parent may not give preventive asthma medicine, even when a child is exhibiting symptoms at the moment.

Individualism and autonomy are highly valued in U.S. culture. People's success is judged by their acquisition of possessions, degrees, and titles. Privacy is also very important. In particular, religion, and spirituality are private matters. On the other hand, in many languages other than English, the word "privacy" does not exist except in the context of "forced isolation." In most other cultures, society is group-oriented. The welfare of the group and cooperation, rather than competition, are primary values in African, Arabic, Asian, and Latino cultures.

Many people from non-Western cultures believe less in their ability to control the future and more in the role of fate. So while Americans tend to "plan and do," focusing on tasks, members of other cultures may tend to "be a part of" and accept their fate.

When working with culturally or spiritually diverse patients and families, we encourage providers to first understand their own cultural values and traditions and to adjust their expectations accordingly. This introduction offers strategies for providers making an initial assessment of the cultural and spiritual needs of a patient and his or her family.

Purpose of the Book

The purpose of this guide is to help health care providers best meet the needs of their patients. To obtain maximum value from this resource, read all of the chapters. Parts One and Two contain samples of beliefs and traditions of various cultural and religious groups. Although readers are encouraged to utilize this material to consider the traditions of the group they serve, they are cautioned not to stereotype or to overgeneralize nor to characterize all members of a cultural or ethnic group as alike. Individuals from the same cultural group may not hold the same values, and a patient's cultural values may or may not be factors in the way the illness is experienced. Aspects to be considered in assessing the situation include: individual characteristics, socioeconomic status, race, education, age, gender, and the stages, conditions, and adjustment to the migration experience, as well as whether the immigrating family lived in a rural or urban area in their native country. The samples are based on one particular hospital's patient population. Other hospitals will have different patient demographics, based on the organization's geographic location. This guide can be used as a template. Using the sample templates provided in Chapter 11, hospitals can write informational material specific to cultural or religious groups in their own patient populations. Chapter 11 also contains information about the use of the interpreter services and the aspects of a bilingual medical interview. Chapter 12 provides tips for meeting the Joint Commission on Accreditation standards related to culture and religion. Some of the Children's Hospital guidelines, including those related to patient ethics, blood transfusions, emergency baptism, and patient and family education, are provided in the Appendix as samples of how policies may be written.

Strategies for Providers

The following information is intended for providers who are initiating a health care relationship with a patient or family. Although this information is useful for all families, it is especially helpful for providers who care for patients and families with cultural beliefs, spiritual traditions, or languages that are unfamiliar to them.

Before Meeting with the Patient and His or Her Family

1. Understand your own cultural values and traditions.

2. Acquire basic knowledge of the cultural values, health beliefs, and nutritional practices of the patient and family.

During Conversation with the Patient and Family

1. Determine the level of comprehension in English, and arrange for an interpreter if needed.

2. Ask how the patient and family members prefer to be addressed.

3. Allow family members to choose their own seating for comfortable personal space and eye contact.

4. Avoid body language that may be offensive or misunderstood, such as sitting too close or looking directly into someone's eyes.

5. Speak directly to the client, even if you are using an interpreter.

6. Choose a speech rate and style that promotes understanding and demonstrates respect for the client.

7. Avoid slang, technical jargon, and complex sentences.

8. Use open-ended questions or questions phrased in several ways to obtain information.

According to Kleinman, Eisenberg, and Good (1978), understanding someone's cultural background assists in the development of an individualized, comprehensive plan of care. Certain questions can help the provider establish a relationship with and exchange important information with the family. The explanatory model of illness posits that a patient interprets and defines symptoms. Using this dialogue, the provider can help the patient understand and communicate his or her feelings about the illness. Kleinman recommends the following sample questions. Document the answers in the patient's record.

Questions to Ask

1. What brings you here (to the hospital, clinic)?

2. What do you call your child's (illness, problem)?

3. What do you think has caused the (illness, problem)?

4. What have (doctors, nurses, other caregivers) done so far? What have you or other family members done so far?

5. How has the illness affected your child's life?

6. How has it affected you and your family?

7. What worries you most about the illness and its treatment?

8. What would you like to have happen today at the clinic/hospital?

During Patient and Family Teaching

1. Determine the patient and family's reading ability before using written material.

2. Review the client's understanding and acceptance of recommendations.

3. Adapt the plan of care as necessary to ensure optimal patient health.

Using the explanatory model of illness, one can elicit information about the individual's beliefs and preferences.

References

American Association of Retired Persons. (1996). Appreciating diversity: A tool for building bridges. Washington, DC: AARP Publications [ww.aarp.org]

Kleinman, A., Eisenberg, L., & Good, B. (1978, February). Culture, illness and care: Clinical lessons from anthropological and cross-cultural research. Annals of Internal Medicine, 88(2), 251–258.

U. S. Department of Agriculture, (1986). Cross-cultural counseling: A guide for nutrition and health counselors. (Report number FNS–250) Washington, DC: USDA.

Part One

Cultural Traditions

Chapter 1
Africa

Cape Verde

Introduction

This information is given as an introduction to a specific culture and is meant to help providers understand similarities and variations in cultural practices. Providers are cautioned not to overgeneralize or characterize all members of a cultural or ethnic group as alike. Factors to be considered in assessing a person's cultural identity and his or her actions or beliefs include individual characteristics, socioeconomic status, race, education, religion, age, gender; the stages, conditions, and adjustment to the migration experience; and whether the family comes from a rural or urban area.

This sheet is specific to Cape Verdean traditions and practices.

Country of Origin and Geographic Location

Cape Verde is an archipelago of nine islands located three hundred miles off the West Coast of Senegal, Africa.

Language

Cape Verdean (Creole) and Portuguese are spoken. Portuguese is the official language; however, most communication is in Cape Verdean, a language based on Portuguese and native dialects.

Migration Patterns

In the late 17th Century, Cape Verde was a regular port of call for American merchant ships in their trade with West Africa. Cape Verdeans came to the United States to work in the whaling industry. Many were eager to leave the islands, which were ravaged by drought and famine. Today, the largest community of Cape Verdeans outside the archipelago lives in Massachusetts. There are also large Cape Verdean communities in Rhode Island and Connecticut. Approximately 400,000 Cape Verdeans live in the United States.

Spiritual Traditions

Most Cape Verdeans are devout Catholics. The church pervades many aspects of the community. Small Protestant denominations are also found, both in the islands and among the immigrants to the United States. In Massachusetts there are established Cape Verdean churches.

Family

Cape Verdeans view the family as the center of their lives. Elders are respected and obeyed. "Women are often considered to be the bedrock of Cape Verdean society, especially in terms of the preservation of linguistic skills, handicrafts, food preparation, and family solidarity" (Lobban, 1996, p. 8). Extended family is important. They are often the first to be consulted in times of illness. Neighbors are often considered as extended family. Hard work, honesty, and respect are very important in the Cape Verdean family circle. Physical punishment, in moderation, is used to discipline children as a last resort. Abusive punishment is not tolerated.

As is the case with many immigrant groups, family and generational tension may arise when children quickly adopt American cultural values that may be in conflict with traditional values.

Diet and Nutrition

"Katxupa" (or "manchupa"), the national dish, is based on dried corn, meat, beans, and vegetables, and can be prepared in many different ways. There are many corn-based dishes in the Cape Verdean diet. Red meat, fried food, dairy products, juice, and sodas are staples of the diet.

Attitudes and General Beliefs About Illness and Death

Serious illness and disability may be seen as God's will. The disabled family member may be protected to the point of isolation. Providers may need to be more active in teaching about the availability of and right to community services and in empowering patients and families to obtain these services.

Implications for Providers

Cultural Courtesies   Behavior outside the home, and in the presence of strangers, tends to be more formal and less expressive as a sign of respect and deference.

Communication Patterns and Value Orientation   In the home and with friends and family, Cape Verdeans are more expressive and emotional.

- Children tend to be dependent on parents. They are expected to be seen and not heard and are taught that information about the family is not to be shared with outsiders. Because children tend to be reserved unless they are with family and trusted friends, having parents in the hospital room may facilitate easier interaction with children.

- Cape Verdeans are generally hard working. They may work many hours, often leaving little time for entertainment. Inflexible work schedules and demands sometimes interfere with parents' ability to visit older children when they are hospitalized.

- Some families may view the hospital bed space as professional space. Parents may be intimidated and hesitate to get close to the patient, seeing their actions as intrusive to patient care.

- The idea of adults playing with children (particularly in a hospital environment) may be foreign, depending on the education and acculturation of the parent. Providers should encourage parents to provide physical and emotional support and take an active part in their child's daily activities.

- During serious illness there is an internal sadness or sense of mourning that may not be easily communicated to others. This sadness may be related to the fact that in Cape Verde, many people die due to illness and poverty.

- When grieving, Cape Verdeans are very expressive and emotionally intense.

- In Cape Verde, wakes take place at home, and funerals are held within twenty-four hours of the death. In the United States, American customs are generally followed, so the funeral may be delayed.

Traditional Medical Practices   "Curanderas" or "curiosas" are lay healers who may be consulted in times of illness. Teas and herbs are prescribed for some conditions. Certain herbs may be burned to ward off evil spirits.

- "Difluxan" is a catch-all term to describe general cold and sinus symptoms, such as itchy, watery eyes, sinus pain, and congestion.
- "Konta d'odju" are amulets with black and white beads. They are given to children soon after birth, or when ill, to ward off evil spirits. They may be pinned on the patient's clothing. Remove these only after discussion with the patient and family.

Other Issues Relevant to Hospitalization   There may be, among some Cape Verdeans, certain beliefs about blood.

- "Sangi durmidu" (sleeping blood), "sangi mortu" (dead blood), or "sange pezode" (bruised blood) is believed to result from a traumatic injury (resulting in a bruise or contusion as defined in Western medicine).
- The "sangi vivu," living blood, leaks out into the skin or becomes deposited in other regions of the body. The blood becomes "sleeping," "dead," or "bruised" and must be removed by either self-treatment in minor cases or surgical removal in more severe cases.
- Some believe that, if this condition is not treated, more serious complications can occur (Like & Ellison, 1981).

References

Like, R., & Ellison, J. (1981). Sleeping blood, tremor and paralysis: A transcultural approach to unusual conversion reaction. *Culture, Medicine and Psychiatry, 5*, 49–63.

Lobban, R. (Summer, 1996). A synthesis of Capeverdean culture and history. *CIMBOA, 3*.

Sanchez, W., & Thomas, D., (1997, Fall/Winter). Disability and health care in the Capeverdean community: Some preliminary findings from service providers. *CIMBOA, 4*.

Eritrea

Introduction

This information is given as an introduction to a specific culture and is meant to help providers understand similarities and variations in cultural practices. Providers are cautioned not to overgeneralize or characterize all members of a cultural or ethnic group as alike. Factors to be considered in assessing a person's cultural identity and his or her actions or beliefs include individual characteristics, socioeconomic status, race, education, religion, age, gender; the stages, conditions, and adjustment to the migration experience; and whether the family came from a rural or urban area.

This sheet is about Eritrean traditions and practices.

Country of Origin and Geographic Location

Eritrea is located on the East Coast of Africa.

Language

The official languages of Eritrea are Tigrinia, Tigrai, and Arabic. Eritreans prefer to be differentiated from Ethiopians, although many speak the same language, Amharic, which is the official language of Ethiopia. Many Eritreans speak English, which is now taught in the schools.

Migration Patterns

In 1962, Ethiopia annexed Eritrea. Eritreans were forced to abandon their separate identity, including their language. In 1991, after twenty-nine years of civil war, Eritrea regained its independence. Many Eritreans sought refuge in other countries during the civil war.

Spiritual Traditions

The two dominant religions are Orthodox (Coptic) and Muslim.

Family

In general, women are considered to be subordinate to men. Girls receive less education than boys do. Families tend to be large by Western standards. Many have seven or eight children. Knowledge and use of family planning may be limited. Family structure includes the extended family. The divorce rate is high. In times of crisis, the extended family may take full responsibility for the family member's problems, whether it is health or finance related. Elders are respected. They are addressed as "aunt" or "uncle," even if they are strangers. Toilet training begins at five to six months of age.

Diet and Nutrition

Eritrean women do not breast-feed for the first twenty-four hours after giving birth. Instead, they give the child sugar water. After the first twenty-four hours, mothers will breast-feed for as long as they wish, often until they are ready to have another child.

Many orthodox Coptic do not eat meat, eggs, or milk on Wednesday or Friday. They also do not eat poultry, beef, or dairy products for fifty-five days before the Easter holiday. Muslims will fast during the daylight hours of Ramadan, which begins either in December or January, depending on the Western calendar, and lasts for one month.

Attitudes and General Beliefs About Illness and Death

Illness may be considered a punishment from God for one's sins or as the anger of the spirits. Mental illness may be considered to be the result of evil spirits, and it is often treated with prayer. Many East Africans have a concept of spirits residing in each individual. When the spirits become angry, illness such as fever, headache, dizziness, and weakness can result. Healing ceremonies are designed to appease the spirits. Many East Africans have a concept of the "evil eye." A person can give someone else an evil eye either purposefully or inadvertently by directing comments of praise at that person, which may cause harm or illness. Mothers may be offended when they hear someone tell them that their child looks big and fat (being heavy or fat is considered a status symbol for adults), out of fear that the evil eye will cause something bad to happen to their child. More acceptable comments are that the child is healthy or beautiful.

Implications for Providers

Cultural Courtesies   The Koran dictates social behavior of Muslims.

- Muslim men and women do not touch one another in public.

- The right hand is considered to be the clean and polite hand to use for daily tasks such as eating, writing, and greeting people. If a child begins to show left-handed preference in writing, he or she will be trained to use his or her right hand.

Communication Patterns and Value Orientation   Health care providers in East Africa are often more personal than the business-like

Western providers. An East African doctor will not inform a patient of a terminal diagnosis. Instead, the doctor will tell a close relative, so that the patient does not become discouraged.

Traditional Medical Practices   Many who come from rural areas depended on traditional healers, who treated illness with herbal and animal remedies. Spiritual healing, such as prayer, is the preferred treatment for many diseases.

- Newborn care includes warm water baths, sesame oil massages, and passive stretching of the baby's limbs.

- In Eritrea, traditional medicine is practiced by older men of the community, who treat conditions such as hepatitis, measles, mumps, chicken pox, "hunch back," facial droop, and broken bones. Treatment may include fire burning, herbal remedies, and prayer. Fire burning is a procedure whereby a stick from a special tree is heated and applied to the skin in order to cure the illness.

- Seizures may be treated with herbs and readings from the Koran.

- Stomachaches, backaches, rashes, and sore throats are often treated with herbs.

- As many as twenty-eight African and Middle Eastern countries, including Eritrea, practice some form of female circumcision. It is also known as female genital mutilation or infibulation. Members of these cultures may believe that removing parts of the vagina, including the clitoris, defines sexual and social identity and promotes the concept of sexual intercourse for procreation only, not allowing for pleasure. Others may believe that the clitoris is the source of illness and that removing it promotes health.

    There are movements and, in some cases, legislation in both East Africa and immigrant communities in the United States to make female circumcision illegal. However, for many women of these cultures, being circumcised promotes socioeconomic survival and cultural identity.

Other Issues Relevant to Hospitalization   Eritreans who consult with doctors usually receive a medication for every illness.

- For those with experience with Western medicine, antibiotics are requested frequently. Because they are accustomed to receiving antibiotics or medications from physicians, they may feel that it is a waste of time to go to a doctor if no medication is given, even for a minor illness.

- Many feel that in Western health care, too much blood is drawn for testing and would prefer it not to be drawn unless absolutely necessary.

- Many who came from rural areas have trouble understanding the Western concept of disease and the causes, means of transmission, and methods of prevention. They also may not understand the practice of withholding treatment until diagnostic work is done.

- Eritrean women may prefer to have an Eritrean woman interpret for them.

References

Compton, K. M., & Chechile, D. (1999). Female genital mutilation. In Kramer and others (Eds.), *Immigrant women's health: Problems and solutions.* San Francisco: Jossey-Bass.

Ethnomed: *www.hslib.washington.edu/clinical/ethnomed/erit.htm*

Ethiopia

Introduction

This information is given as an introduction to a specific culture and is meant to help providers understand similarities and variations in cultural practices. Providers are cautioned not to overgeneralize or characterize all members of a cultural or ethnic group as alike. Factors to be considered in assessing a person's cultural identity and his or her actions or beliefs include individual characteristics, socioeconomic status, race, education, religion, age, gender; the stages, conditions, and adjustment to the migration experience; and whether the family came from a rural or urban area.

This sheet is about Ethiopian traditions and practices.

Country of Origin and Geographic Location

Ethiopia is located on the East Coast of Africa.

Language

Ethiopians may speak any one of eighty dialects; however, many speak Amharic.

Migration Patterns

Many have left the country since the establishment of a repressive regime in the mid-1970s and subsequent political turmoil in East Africa.

Spiritual Traditions

The two dominant religions are Orthodox (Coptic) and Muslim.

Family

In general, women are considered to be subordinate to men. Girls receive less education than boys do. Families tend to be large; many have seven or eight children. Knowledge and use of family planning may be limited. Family structure includes the extended family. The divorce rate is high. In times of crisis, the extended family may take full responsibility for the family member's problems, whether it is health or finance related. Elders are respected. They are addressed as "aunt" or "uncle," even if they are strangers. Toilet training often begins at five to six months of age.

Diet and Nutrition

Most women breast-feed their babies. They breast-feed for as long as they wish, often until they are ready to have another child.

Many orthodox Coptic do not eat meat, eggs, or milk on Wednesday or Friday. They also do not eat poultry, beef, or dairy products for fifty-five days before the Easter holiday. Muslims fast during the daylight hours of Ramadan, which begins in December or January, depending on the Western calendar, and continues for a month.

Attitudes and General Beliefs About Illness and Death

Illness is often considered a punishment from God for a person's sins or as the anger of the spirits. Mental illness may be considered to be the result of evil spirits, and it is often treated with prayer. Many East Africans have a concept of spirits residing in each individual. When the spirits become angry, illness such as fever, headache, dizziness, and weakness can result. Healing ceremonies are designed to appease the spirits.

Many East Africans also have a concept of the "evil eye." A person can give someone else an evil eye either purposefully or inadvertently by directing comments of praise at that person, which may cause harm or illness. In East Africa, being heavy or fat is considered a status symbol for adults. But mothers may be offended when they hear someone tell them that their child looks big and fat out of fear that the evil eye will cause something bad to happen to their child. More acceptable comments are that the child is healthy or beautiful.

Implications for Providers

Cultural Courtesies   The majority of Ethiopians greet people by bowing their heads.

- Elders and men in positions of status may shake hands using both hands, as a sign of respect.

- The right hand is considered to be the clean and polite hand to use for daily tasks such as eating, writing, and greeting people.

- If a child begins to show left-handed preference, he or she will be trained to use his or her right hand.

- Ethiopian men and women who are Muslim do not touch one another in public.

Communication Patterns and Value Orientation   Health care providers in East Africa are often more personal than the business-like Western providers.

- In Ethiopia, a doctor will not inform a patient of a terminal diagnosis. Instead, the doctor will tell a close relative, so that the patient does not become discouraged.

- Ethiopians have no middle name, only a first and last name.

Traditional Medical Practices   Many who come from rural areas have used traditional healers, who treat illness with herbal and animal remedies. Spiritual healing, such as prayer, is the preferred treatment for many diseases.

- Newborn care may include warm water baths, sesame oil massages, and passive stretching of the baby's limbs.

- In Ethiopia, traditional medicine is often practiced by older men of the community, who treat conditions such as hepatitis, measles, mumps, chicken pox, hunch back, facial droop, and broken bones. Treatment may include fire burning, herbal remedies, and prayer, as well as casting of broken bones. Fire burning is a procedure whereby a stick from a special tree is heated and applied to the skin in order to cure an illness. Seizures may be treated with herbs and readings from the Koran. Stomachaches, backaches, rashes, and sore throats are often treated with herbs.

- As many as twenty-eight African and Middle-Eastern countries, including Ethiopia, practice some form of female circumcision. It is also known as female genital mutilation or infibulation. Many believe that removing parts of the vagina, including the clitoris, defines sexual and social identity and promotes the concept of sexual intercourse for procreation only, not allowing for pleasure. Others may believe that the clitoris is the source of illness and that removing it promotes health.

  There are movements and, in some cases, legislation in both East Africa and immigrant communities in the United States to make female circumcision illegal. However, for many women of these cultures, being circumcised promotes socioeconomic survival and cultural identity. Most women who have had exposure to Western medicine understand that female circumcision is not practiced in the United States.

Other Issues Relevant to Hospitalization   Many who came from rural areas in East Africa may have trouble understanding the Western concept of disease and the causes, means of transmission, and methods of prevention.

- East Africans may not understand the practice of withholding treatment until diagnostic work is done. Because many go to a doctor believing that the primary reason for doing so is to receive antibiotics or medication, they may imply that it is a waste of time to go to a doctor if no medication is given, even for a minor illness.

- When a person is considered terminally ill, it is considered uncaring for a physician to tell the patient that he or she is dying.

- Ethiopians often spank their children when they misbehave. In East African culture, spanking is not considered abusive.

References

Compton, K. M., & Chechile, D. (1999). Female genital mutilation. In Kramer and others (Eds.), *Immigrant women's health: Problems and solutions.* San Francisco: Jossey-Bass.

Molakign, A. (1996). Ethnomed: *www.hslib.washington.edu/clinical/ethnomed/ethiopcp.htm*

Nigeria

Introduction

This information is given as an introduction to a specific culture and is meant to help providers understand similarities and variations in cultural practices. Providers are cautioned not to overgeneralize or characterize all members of a cultural or ethnic group as alike. Factors to be considered in assessing a person's cultural identity and his or her actions or beliefs include individual characteristics, socioeconomic status, race, education, religion, age, gender; the stages, conditions, and adjustment to the migration experience; and whether the family came from a rural or urban area.

This sheet is about the Nigerian tradition and practices.

Country of Origin and Geographic Location

Nigeria is located in West Africa, on the Atlantic Ocean. It is the most densely populated country in Africa.

Language

There are more than 250 languages spoken in Nigeria. Because it was once colonized, the official language of Nigeria is English; however, less than half the population speaks the language. A larger percentage speaks "broken English." There are about 532 ethnic groups (also known as "tribes") in Nigeria. The three primary ethnic groups and their languages are Hausa, Yoruba, and Ibo. Many Nigerians speak more than one language.

Migration Patterns

Many Nigerians come to the United States for educational and economic opportunities or to avoid political conflict in West Africa.

Spiritual Traditions

Most Nigerians are practicing Muslims or Christians. The Hausa come from the northern part of Nigeria and are predominantly Muslim. The Ibo come from the southern part of the country and are predominantly Christian. The Yoruba may be Christian or Muslim. Some follow traditional African belief systems.

Family

Nigerian families tend to be close-knit, including extended families. It is common for grandparents to live with their children and grandchildren. Often people are accorded respect on the basis of their family's collective achievements and not on one member's status or position in society.

Nigerian fathers tend to be the primary decision makers. It is important to include the eldest man in all decision making.

Islamic law allows Muslim men to have more than one wife. Nigerian children are brought up to respect parents, other family members, and their elders. Parents begin to discipline their children at an early age. Spanking is accepted in Nigerian culture. It is allowed in schools as a way for teachers to discipline students.

Diet and Nutrition

Most Nigerians enjoy hot, spicy food. The main staples of the Nigerian diet are starches: yams, "cassava" (a starchy, root vegetable), beans, and rice. Meals may include fish, meat, or chicken, in a pepper sauce. Some Nigerians tend to eat with their hands (right hand only), while others use utensils. Nigerians who are Muslim follow the dietary proscriptions of Islam.

Attitudes and General Beliefs About Illness and Death

Although a public health care system exists in many African countries, health care is largely unavailable for people who are poor and living in rural areas. Most children in Nigeria have had basic immunizations but very little primary care. Because parents tend to project hope for the future to their children, many will seek out primary care once in the United States. Some West Africans believe that illness may be caused by behavior, for example, someone who lies or physically hurts another person may become sick as punishment for his or her actions.

Nigerians tend to rely on their extended family and friends for support during the illness and death of a family member. Many traditions revolve around the religious beliefs of the family.

Implications for Providers

Cultural Courtesies   Different cultural groups, tribes, and generations have distinct beliefs about appropriate behavior. However, the following examples usually apply to most Nigerians.

- It is generally considered appropriate to bow one's head when greeting.
- It is important to take time to greet a Nigerian and not to rush through the process, as rushing is considered rude and disrespectful.

- It is customary to shake hands when greeting. When people know one another well, kissing each other on each cheek is common.

- It is common for friends of the same sex to hold hands or hug.

- Nigerians usually pass objects with either the right hand or both hands. It is considered rude to pass objects with the left hand alone, especially to an elder.

- It is important not to display the palm of the hand, with the fingers spread out, or the sole of the foot. Both are considered disrespectful.

Communication Patterns and Value Orientation   Because there are so many different tribes in Nigeria, communication patterns and value orientation patterns differ. But all tribes have some communication patterns and values in common, such as:

- Personal space between members of the same sex is very limited. Nigerians tend to stand or sit very close to others when conversing.

- Doctors in Nigeria will discuss the seriousness of an illness with the next of kin. It is bad luck to tell the patient.

- West Africans are taught to respect authority figures. They may not contradict or question a health care provider. However, this does not mean that they necessarily intend to comply with the prescribed care plan.

Traditional Medical Practices   Many Nigerians may practice Western medicine, yet rely on a traditional healer or native doctor as well. Nearly every village in Nigeria has a healer.

- Many treatments used by traditional healers come from extracts of roots, herbs, tree bark, and leaves.

- Belief in the "evil eye" is common for many Nigerians. One might wear an amulet, a rope, or a leather strap for protection.

References

David Kennedy Center for International Studies. (1996). *Culturgrams: Nigeria.* Provo, UT: Brigham Young University.

New York Task Force on Immigrant Health. (1997). *Health beliefs and practices of West African immigrants.* New York: New York University School of Medicine.

Somalia

Introduction

This information is given as an introduction to a specific culture and is meant to help providers understand similarities and variations in cultural practices. Providers are cautioned not to overgeneralize or characterize all members of a cultural or ethnic group as alike. Factors to be considered in assessing a person's cultural identity and his or her actions or beliefs include individual characteristics, socioeconomic status, race, education, religion, age, gender; the stages, conditions, and adjustment to the migration experience; and whether the family came from a rural or urban area.

This sheet is about Somali traditions and practices.

Country of Origin and Geographic Location

Somalia is located on the East Coast of Africa.

Language

The primary language in Somalia is Somali. The vast majority of Somali are Muslim, and so the second language for many is Arabic.

Migration Patterns

In 1991, people began to leave Somalia to escape wars between inter-clans or tribes and the subsequent famine and disaster. Resettlement programs have enabled families to move to the United States.

Spiritual Traditions

Almost all Somalis are Sunni Muslims. Many attitudes, social customs, and gender roles are primarily based on Islamic tradition.

Family

In general, women are considered to be subordinate to men. Girls receive less education than boys do. Families tend to be large; many have seven or eight children. Knowledge and use of family planning may be limited. Family structure includes the extended family. The divorce rate is high. In times of crisis, the extended family may take full responsibility for the family member's problems, whether it is health or finance related. Elders are respected. They are addressed as "aunt" or "uncle," even if they are strangers.

Diet and Nutrition

Muslims fast during the daylight hours of Ramadan, which begins in late December and early January, depending on the Western calendar, and lasts for one month. It is common to breast-feed infants up to two years of age.

Attitudes and General Beliefs About Illness and Death

Illness may be considered a punishment from God for a person's sins or as a sign of the anger of the spirits. Mental illness is considered to be the result of evil spirits and is treated with prayer. Many East Africans have a concept of spirits residing in each individual. When the spirits become angry, illness such as fever, headache, dizziness, and weakness can result. Healing ceremonies are designed to appease the spirits. Many East Africans have a concept of the "evil eye." A person can give someone else an evil eye, either purposefully or inadvertently, by directing comments of praise at that person, which may cause harm or illness. Somali mothers may be offended when they hear someone tell them that their child looks big and fat out of fear that the evil eye will cause something bad to happen to their child. More acceptable comments are that the child is healthy or beautiful.

Implications for Providers

Cultural Courtesies   Somali names have three parts: the first name is the given name, the second is the name of the father, and the third is the name of the paternal grandfather. Male and female siblings will share the second and third names. Women, when they marry, do not change their names.

- The right hand is considered to be the clean and polite hand to use for daily tasks such as eating, writing, and greeting people.
- If a child begins to show left-handed preference, the child will be trained to use his or her right hand.
- Muslim men and women do not touch one another in public.

Communication Patterns and Value Orientation   Health care providers in East Africa are more personal than are business-like Western providers. An East African doctor will not inform a patient of a terminal diagnosis. Instead, the doctor will tell a close relative, so that the patient does not become discouraged.

Traditional Medical Practices   Many who come from rural areas depended on traditional healers, who treated illness with herbal and animal remedies.

- Spiritual healing, such as prayer, is the preferred treatment for many diseases.

- In Somalia, traditional medicine is practiced by older men of the community, who treat conditions such as hepatitis, measles, mumps, chicken pox, hunch back, facial droop, and broken bones. Treatment includes fire burning, herbal remedies, and prayer.

- Fire burning is a procedure whereby a stick from a special tree is heated and applied to the skin in order to cure the illness.

- Seizures may be treated with herbs and readings from the Koran.

- Stomachaches, backaches, rashes, and sore throats are treated with herbs.

- Newborn care includes warm water baths, sesame oil massages, and passive stretching of the baby's limbs.

- When a child is born, the new mother and baby stay indoors at home for forty days, a time period known as "afatanbah." During the afatanbah, the mother may wear earrings made from string placed through a clove of garlic and the baby may wear a bracelet made from string and herbs, in order to ward off the evil eye.

- As many as twenty-eight African and Middle-Eastern countries, including Somalia, practice some form of female circumcision. It is also known as female genital mutilation or infibulation. Many believe that removing parts of the vagina, including the clitoris, defines sexual and social identity and promotes the concept of sexual intercourse for procreation only, not allowing for pleasure. Others may believe that the clitoris is the source of illness and that removing it promotes health. Female circumcision is usually performed between birth and five years of age.

   There are movements and, in some cases, legislation in both East Africa and immigrant communities in the United States to make female circumcision illegal. However, for many women of these cultures, being circumcised promotes socioeconomic survival and cultural identity. Most women who have had exposure to Western medicine understand that female circumcision is not practiced in the United States.

Other Issues Relevant to Hospitalization   Many who came from rural areas of East Africa may have trouble understanding the Western concept of disease and the causes, means of transmission, and methods of prevention.

- East Africans may not understand the practice of withholding treatment until diagnostic work is done. Because many go to a doctor believing that the primary reason for doing so is to receive antibiotics or medication, they may imply that it is a waste of time to go to a doctor if no medication is given, even for a minor illness.

- When a person is considered terminally ill, it is considered uncaring for a physician to tell the patient or family that the person is dying.

References

Compton, K. M., & Chechile, D. (1999). Female genital mutilation. In Kramer and others (Eds.), *Immigrant women's health: Problems and solutions.* San Francisco: Jossey-Bass.

Ethnomed: *www.hslib.washington.edu/clinical/ethnomed/somali.htm*

Lewis, T., Hussein, K., Ahmed, K., Ahmed, B, & Mohammed, A. (1996). *Somali families.* Seattle, WA: University of Washington, Healthlinks.

Chapter 2

Asia

Cambodia

Introduction

This information is given as an introduction to a specific culture and is meant to help providers understand similarities and variations in cultural practices. Providers are cautioned not to overgeneralize or characterize all members of a cultural or ethnic group as alike. Factors to be considered in assessing a person's cultural identity and his or her actions or beliefs include individual characteristics, socioeconomic status, race, education, religion, age, gender; the stages, conditions, and adjustment to the migration experience; and whether the family came from a rural or urban area.

This sheet is about Cambodian traditions and practices.

Country of Origin and Geographic Location

Cambodia is part of Southeast Asia, also known as Indochina, on the Malay Peninsula.

Language

Cambodian or Khmer

Migration Patterns

During the Vietnam War, Cambodia was the target of many attacks. A civil war in Cambodia followed. By 1975, the Khmer Rouge regime, lead by Pol Pot, took power. Cambodians suffered tremendous hardship under this dictatorship. In 1979, the Vietnamese troops invaded Cambodia and installed a new Vietnamese Communist government. As a result, Cambodians began to escape from their homeland to refugee camps in Thailand. Many subsequently came to the United States. Many Cambodian immigrants have experienced tremendous stress associated with their departure. They may have suffered from psychological and physical ailments, as well as the trauma of loss of and separation from family members.

Spiritual Traditions

Eighty-five percent of Cambodians are Buddhist. The other 15 percent are Muslim or Christian. Many believe in the power of the supernatural. During the Communist regimes, expression of religion was prohibited.

Family

The husband is considered to be the primary decision maker in the family. Children are initially perceived as relatively helpless and not responsible for their actions; therefore, Southeast Asian parents always remind their children of their behavior, focusing on modeling rather than the use of strict discipline. Mother-infant interaction is characterized by an emphasis on close physical contact. Toilet training may be introduced as early as three months of age.

Diet and Nutrition

In Cambodia there are two basic dishes: soup and white rice. Many Southeast Asians dislike milk and consume it infrequently; many Southeast Asians are also lactose-intolerant. Food preferences are commonly practiced during an illness. Cambodians may avoid beef, chicken, bamboo shoots, peanuts, and eggplant when they have a skin disease.

Attitudes and General Beliefs About Illness and Death

Health care in Southeast Asia tends to be reactive, based on relief of symptoms. Prevention seems to be less of a priority. During the time of illness, traditional rituals and prayers are held in the home. Some may believe that illness is a punishment for faults. In many cases, the deceased are bathed and dressed in new clothes, and a coin is inserted in the mouth. A religious ceremony, known as "Prachum Ben," recalls the spirit of dead people. It takes place in September. It is a time for children to offer food to Buddha to release the sins of ancestors so that they may pass to a better life.

Implications for Providers

Cultural Courtesies   Some rules regarding gestures originate from Buddhist practice.

- When seated, the provider should not point his or her feet toward the client, as the feet are considered to be the most inferior part of the body. The head is the most sacred.

- The provider should not touch the patient's head, if possible, or should do so only with warning.

- The provider should avoid sitting or standing on a level more elevated than that of an elder.

- To show respect, many Southeast Asians will bow their heads to a superior or elder.

- In conversation, respect is shown by avoiding direct eye contact.

- Women do not shake hands with one another or with men.

Communication Patterns and Value Orientation   Many values are based on both the Confucian respect for education, family, and elders, and the Taoist desire to avoid conflict.

- Sparing one's feelings is considered more important than factual truth.

- To avoid confrontation or disrespect, many will not verbalize disagreement. Instead they may avoid answering the question.

- A smile should not be interpreted as happiness or agreement.

- Speaking in a loud tone with excessive gestures is considered rude, especially when done by women.

- Silence is welcomed and in most situations more appropriate than "small talk."

- Summoning a person with a hand or finger in the upright position is considered derogatory. To summon a person, the entire hand with the fingers facing down is the only appropriate hand signal.

Traditional Medical Practices   Many Southeast Asian traditional medical practices are derived from Chinese medicine. This system is based on the premise that living things are composed of five basic elements: air, fire, water, earth, and metal. The associated characteristics are cold, hot, wet, and dry, and one's body must maintain proper balance to be healthy.

- The theory of illness is also based on the yin/yang or cold/hot classification of various diseases.

- Dermabrasive procedures based on hot/cold physiology are often used to treat coughs and other maladies. Cutaneous hematomas are made over the face, neck, and trunk to release air. These are made in many different ways: by pinching and pulling on the skin, by rubbing oiled skin with the edge of a coin or spoon, or by cupping. Cupping is done by heating the air in a cup with a flame, then placing the cup onto the skin.

- Tiger balm is often used for headaches, nausea, and muscle aches.

Other Issues Relevant to Hospitalization   Among middle-aged and older Cambodians, there may be discomfort with giving written consent. During the civil war, signed life histories were required from individuals who were later executed.

- Providers are advised to translate consent forms using a Cambodian interpreter, who will ensure understanding. Mental health issues are often interpreted differently than in the Western medical system.

- Mental problems are often believed to be caused by supernatural spirits, strain on the mind, or other psychosocial issues. Treatment is sought from family members, elders, or healers in the community.

- Most Cambodians do not celebrate birthdays. Many celebrate the Cambodian New Year, which is a very important three-day festival in mid-April.

References

Kulig, J. (1996). Cambodian culture. In J. G.. Lipson, S. L. Dibble, & P. A. Minarik (Eds.), *Culture & nursing care: A pocket guide.* San Francisco, CA: University of California San Francisco Nursing Press.

Lynch, E. W., & Hanson, M. J. (1992). *Developing cross-cultural competence.* Baltimore, MD: Paul H. Brookes Publishing.

Office of Refugee and Immigrant Health. (1995). *Refugees and immigrants in Massachusetts: An overview of selected communities.* Boston, MA: Bureau of Family and Community Health and the Massachusetts Department of Public Health.

China

Introduction

This information is given as an introduction to a specific culture and is meant to help providers understand similarities and variations in cultural practices. Providers are cautioned not to overgeneralize or characterize all members of a cultural or ethnic group as alike. Factors to be considered in assessing a person's cultural identity and his or her actions or beliefs include individual characteristics, socioeconomic status, race, education, religion, age, gender; the stages, conditions, and adjustment to the migration experience; and whether the family came from a rural or urban area.

This sheet is about Chinese traditions and practices.

Country of Origin and Geographic Location

People's Republic of China ("mainland China"), Hong Kong, and Taiwan.

Language

Mandarin Chinese is spoken by more than 70 percent of the population of the People's Republic of China and Taiwan. Chinese who immigrated from Hong Kong and Southeast China speak Cantonese. Other regional and local Chinese dialects are also spoken. All dialects of spoken Chinese share the same written language (Mandarin).

Migration Patterns

In the 1800s, many Chinese immigrated to the United States to escape widespread famine, economic depression, and civil war. Racism in America resulted in the Chinese Exclusion Act of 1882 that banned any Chinese from entering the country until 1942. In 1965, a new law abolished immigration quotas, and a second wave of urban, educated Chinese professionals and skilled workers settled, primarily in California and New York. Since the 1980s, many scholars have chosen to stay in the United States after completing their studies or have left China to avoid recent political problems.

Spiritual Traditions

Older generations may be influenced by a blend of Buddhism, Taoism, and Confucianism. A small minority of Chinese are Muslim or Christian. Many Chinese will say they have no particular religious tradition, although they may be active spiritually.

Family

Family is considered to be the foundation of Chinese society. Family includes multiple generations, as well as an active inclusion of ancestors in daily life. Immediate family typically includes the husband, wife, unmarried children, married sons, daughters-in-law, and grandchildren. The most treasured values of Chinese society are expressed in family relationships: loyalty, obligation, obedience, cooperation, interdependence, and reciprocity (Lynch & Hanson, 1992). The father is typically the family spokesperson and decision maker in the public domain, and the mother is the manager of the house, child rearing, and finances. Children may sleep in the parental bed until school age and may breast feed up to age two or longer. Children are often completely toilet trained as early as one year of age.

Diet and Nutrition

Many prefer traditional Chinese cooking to a Western diet. A hospitalized child may be unfamiliar with items on the hospital menu, and staff may encourage the parents to bring more familiar foods from home to increase intake. "Congee" is rice porridge given to sick children.

Attitudes and General Beliefs About Illness and Death

In Chinese culture, physical problems are not easily separated from psychological or spiritual concerns. Illness may be seen as caused by spirits, by improper emotions, or by taboo behaviors, in addition to typical scientific causes. Disability can carry a stigma, as it is sometimes associated with bad luck or inappropriate prenatal behavior of the birth mother.

The attitude of the ill person may vary according to religious belief or nonbelief. Alertness up to the time of death may be spiritually important, and the patient or family may refuse pain relief if it is believed to impair consciousness. In general, Chinese do not readily report discomfort.

Family members may not tell the patient that he or she is dying and may not discuss it with one another. Younger generations may be more open to talking about a patient's illness and may wish to know the prognosis. It may be important for family members to be present at the time of death. There is concern for the care and image of the body. The women in the family prepare special funeral clothes. Funerals are elaborate and rich with tradition.

Implications for Providers

Cultural Courtesies   Chinese names typically consist of a one-syllable family name, followed by a one-syllable or two-syllable first name. A person is addressed by his or her full name or by a title with a family name. For example, Lu La Mei may be addressed as Mrs. Lu. Chinese children living in the United States may have both an American and a Chinese first name.

- When one Chinese helps another, the one who receives help owes a debt of gratitude to the helper. That debt may be repaid in a gift or an invitation to a family event.

- A provider's reluctance to accept a family's gift or invitation may be misconstrued as insulting.

Communication Patterns and Value Orientation   In China, one usually avoids saying "no" out of respect to the other person. Chinese people typically communicate more with the use of nonverbal language, and may be saying "yes" when they really mean "no." An interpreter may be able to assist with the clarification of the implied message.

- Chinese persons may see discussing family-related problems with a stranger as potentially disrespectful to their family.

- Beginning a conversation with an attempt at direct problem solving may be counterproductive. Care should be taken to develop a rapport with the family, to allow for seemingly tangential conversation, and to approach the problem at hand in an indirect way.

- Silence in a conversation typically has meaning: an expression of respect, interest, anger, or disagreement. The assistance of an interpreter in clarifying the silence is often helpful.

- Eye contact and casual smiling when speaking with a stranger or person of authority is usually considered disrespectful. A family may be listening attentively even though their affect appears enigmatic or flat.

- Asians typically prefer a greater amount of physical space than North Americans may be accustomed to. Physical touching or displays of affection are uncommon. It would be considered inappropriate to hug or console a Chinese adult or child with touch.

- The American hand gesture for waving good-bye approximates the Chinese gesture for "come here." The typical American beckoning gesture (palm up) should be avoided, because it is considered rude.

Traditional Medical Practices   Ancient China developed a sophisticated medical tradition that included acupuncture, complex herbal medications, and acupressure, as well as sophisticated techniques of diagnosis.

- Many Chinese living in America will follow Western medical advice at the time of illness, but may also seek concurrent traditional herbal treatments or acupuncture.

- One form of traditional medicine includes dermabrasion, which can produce welts and superficial bruises and can easily be mistaken as a sign of physical abuse.

Other Issues Relevant to Hospitalization   Many Chinese workers are employed in small family-owned businesses in which affordable health insurance is unavailable. Preventive and routine health care may be limited.

References

Council of Churches of Greater Springfield and the Visiting Nurse Hospice of Pioneer Valley. (1995). *Knowing my neighbor: Religious beliefs and cultural traditions at times of illness and death.* Springfield, MA: Council of Churches.

Lynch, E. W., & Hanson, M. J. (Eds.). (1992). *Developing cross-cultural competence.* Baltimore, MD: Paul H. Brookes Publishing.

Office of Refugee and Immigrant Health. (1995). *Refugees and immigrants in Massachusetts: An overview of selected communities.* Boston, MA: Bureau of Family and Community Health and the Massachusetts Department of Public Health.

Websites: *www.mic.ki.se/china/html* and *www.wayne.edu/shiffman/altmed/china*

India

Introduction

This information is given as an introduction to a specific culture and is meant to help providers understand similarities and variations in cultural practices. Providers are cautioned not to overgeneralize or characterize all members of a cultural or ethnic group as alike. Factors to be considered in assessing a person's cultural identity and his or her actions or beliefs include individual characteristics, socioeconomic status, race, education, religion, age, gender; the stages, conditions, and adjustment to the migration experience; and whether the family came from a rural or urban area.

The following information is specific to Asian Indian traditions and practices.

Country of Origin and Geographic Location

India is part of Southern Asia. It borders Pakistan, China, Nepal, Sri Lanka, Bhutan, and Bangladesh.

Language

In India, there are at least seventeen recognized languages. The most common languages are Hindi (understood by 71 percent) and English (understood by 31 percent). Other languages include Bengali, Telegu, Marathi, Tamil, Urdu, Gujarati, Malayalam, Kannada, Oriya, Punjabi, Assamese, Kashmiri, Sindhi, Sanskrit, and Hindustani. English is commonly used for national, political, and commercial needs. Many have learned "British English," as Britain ruled India for more than one hundred years, until 1947. Their English vocabulary may be different from that which North Americans use.

Migration Patterns

Most Indian nationals come to the United States for economic or educational reasons. Some come to the United States for business. On average, immigrants and visitors to the United States from India are more educated and affluent than most other Indians are. Emigrés usually maintain close ties with friends and family in India.

Spiritual Traditions

Hinduism and Muslim are the two primary religions. Others include Sikh, Buddhism, Jainism, and Judaism.

Family

Indian families are generally larger than families in the United States. Extended families may live in the same house or close together, and members help out with child care. It would be important for the provider to include the child care provider in discussions about home care. Often marriages in India are arranged, with parents of both the bride and groom more directly involved in choosing and recommending partners than in the United States.

Diet and Nutrition

Many Indians are vegetarians. Most Hindus follow the dietary restrictions of the religion, which prohibits consumption of beef. Some Hindus and Muslims fast during certain times of the year. Traditionally, honey may be given to newborns. Mothers in the United States are cautioned against giving honey because of the high risk of bacterial contamination.

Attitudes and General Beliefs About Illness and Death

Most Indians in the United States understand and accept the Western basics of science, how infectious disease is spread, and how medications can be used to treat disease.

The traditional philosophy and science of medicine in India is called "Ayurveda." "Ayur" means longevity and "veda" means science. It promotes a positive attitude toward health and a daily routine in which diet, hygiene, work, and rest patterns are in sync, as are the body and the five elements of the universe (the five elements are water, fire, earth, wind, and ether). Three of the elements correspond to the elements in the body. These elements are also known as humors: bile (analogous to fire), phlegm (water), and gas or wind (wind). When these elements are in balance, the body is healthy. When the balance is upset, illness results. Consuming certain foods can cause a temperature imbalance. For example, curd, yogurt, fruit, and rice are considered cold, while teas, chicken, garlic, and cloves are hot. Hot and cold do not refer to the spiciness or temperature of the food or one's body, but rather to certain properties of the food. Ayurvedic providers are known as "Vaidyas." Ayurvedic medical schools in India continue to train in and teach these traditions (Butte, 1998).

In India, although all have access to a public health system, most educated and middle class Indians use a fee-for-service private system. There is no concept of health insurance in India.

Implications for Providers

Cultural Courtesies   Traditionally, Indians were divided into castes; an individual belonged to the caste of his or her parents. Belonging to a caste had many implications in terms of career, education, and social standing. Although the caste system has long been considered illegal, discrimination is still present. Indians would rather their sons or daughters marry within the familiar confines of caste, region, and religion (Butte, 1998).

- In India, one smiles only in informal situations, and smiles are exchanged only between those of equal social status.

- Indians may shake their head from side to side to mean "yes."

- Couples express love and affection only in privacy.

- Beckoning is done with the palm turned down, and pointing is considered rude.

Communication Patterns and Value Orientation   India is the largest democracy in the world. Although tolerance and diversity are central to Indian culture, there are recent trends toward nationalism within India. India and Pakistan have had a long-standing territorial dispute over the northern Kashmir region, where religious clashes between Indian Hindus and Pakistani Muslims are not uncommon.

Traditional Medical Practices   In India, colostrum is often believed to be bad for newborns. Sugar water is fed to the baby until the mother's ritual bath on the third day postpartum.

Other Issues Relevant to Hospitalization   Many Indians perceive blood to be precious and not to be wasted. They may hesitate to have blood drawn.

References

Almeida, R. (1996). Indian families. In M. McGoldrick, J. Giordano, & J. K. Pearce (Eds.), *Ethnicity and family therapy* (2nd ed.). New York: Guilford Press.

Butte, A. (1998). Private conversations. Boston, MA; Children's Hospital.

CIA World Fact Book: *www.odci.gov/cia/publications/factbook/country-frame. html*

Ramakrishna, J., & Weiss, M. (1992, September). Health, illness and immigration—East Indians in the United States: Cross-cultural medicine a decade later. *Western Journal of Medicine, 157,* 265–270.

Website: *www.mic.ki.se/india/html*

Japan

Introduction

This information is given as an introduction to a specific culture and is meant to help providers understand similarities and variations in cultural practices. Providers are cautioned not to overgeneralize or characterize all members of a cultural or ethnic group as alike. Factors to be considered in assessing a person's cultural identity and his or her actions or beliefs include individual characteristics, socioeconomic status, race, education, religion, age, gender; the stages, conditions, and adjustment to the migration experience; and whether the family came from a rural or urban area.

The following information is about Japanese traditions and practices.

Country of Origin and Geographic Location

Japan is located in the Pacific Ocean. The country is composed of four large islands—Hokkaido, Honshu, Shikoku, and Kyushu—and approximately four thousand small islands.

Language

Japanese is spoken.

Migration Patterns

All Asians were prohibited from entering the United States between 1924 and 1950. Japanese immigrants who arrived before 1924 created self-contained communities along the West Coast of the United States. By isolating themselves from the prejudice of Caucasian Americans, these communities were able to retain their cultural traditions and values. In 1942, as a result of World War II, anyone of Japanese ancestry living on the Pacific Coast was put in a relocation camp. Survivors of this treatment may have internalized their feelings related to the experience and not shared them with their children. Immigration was renewed in 1950. Many Japanese are temporarily in the United States to study or work in companies bought by Japanese corporations.

Spiritual Traditions

Many Japanese claim not to be very religious. Many practice a mix of Buddhism, Shinto (ancient Japanese tradition), and Confucianism. Some second-generation Japanese-Americans practice Christianity. Many Japanese celebrate Christmas and Oshogatsu, the Japanese New Year.

Family

Japanese immigrants use titles to describe the generation in which they were born and to describe age, experience, language, and values. "Issei" are the first generation to live in the United States. "Nissei" are the second generation of Japanese-Americans to live in the United States, but the first to be U.S. born. "Sansei" are third generation (most are in their 40s and 50s), followed by "Yonsei" (fourth). Sansei and Yonsei are relatively indistinguishable from other Americans in both traditions and values. In most traditional families, respect is the primary value. This can be reflected in their interactions with others, particularly elders. Japanese society tends to be patriarchal: fathers are the primary decision makers, whereas mothers are the primary caretakers. In the past, sons were valued more than daughters. Parents tend to be permissive with children, as they are revered. Until the age of five or six, children are taught by example rather than through verbal rules or punishment. Japanese children sleep with parents, often until they are school age. Breast-feeding may continue until the children are about three years old.

Diet and Nutrition

Primary staples of the traditional Japanese diet are fish, soybean protein (tofu), rice, noodles, and vegetables. They are typically served in small dishes rather than on one large plate. It is important to have a meal that is visually appealing. Many Asians are lactose intolerant and therefore avoid milk products. Rice porridge is often given to Japanese children when they are ill. Some children are given "umeboshi" plum with hot tea or rice. Some use "gen-mai-cha" (tea with puffed rice) for stomach ailments.

Attitudes and General Beliefs About Illness and Death

Japanese express the importance of harmony and balance among themselves, society, and the universe. Disease is seen as an imbalance or disharmony. Those who practice Shinto may believe that disease is caused by an impurity caused by the evil of external forces or spirits. The Kampo medical belief posits that wellness is a balance of the forces of nature; therefore, an imbalance would cause illness. These theories are very different from Western biomedical theory, which views disease as a biological imbalance. Providers are encouraged to keep this in mind when explaining the cause of a patient's illness.

Implications for Providers

Cultural Courtesies   As with all adults, providers should use last names when greeting patients. It may be considered insulting to use first names only.

- Older generations greet one another with a smile and a small bow. Younger generations (Japanese-Americans) greet others with a handshake.

- Direct eye contact is often considered disrespectful, primarily with older generations.

- Physical space is important; providers who must touch the patient should ask permission first.

- Privacy and modesty are important parts of Japanese culture. If possible, patient and provider should be of the same gender.

Communication Patterns and Value Orientation   In communication, importance is placed on attitude, actions, and feelings, rather than on the words. Constant talk is considered unnecessary. An overly talkative or "chatty" person may be considered insincere.

- Overt conflict is minimized both in and outside the home. It is generally considered impolite to express disagreement, particularly with elders.

- Control of emotions is considered important. The concepts of self-restraint and the ability to endure stress are paramount. Often patients may appear stoic or unemotional in their reaction to painful procedures. The concept of "saving face" is pervasive throughout the Japanese culture.

- One usually does not say "no" or disagree with providers. The patient may be saying "yes" or nodding the head when he or she really means "no." An interpreter may be able to assist with the clarification of the implied message.

- The use of mental health services may be considered shameful to the family. One might describe an emotional conflict by complaining about a physical ailment.

Traditional Medical Practices   The Kampo medical belief endorses the use of particular foods as preventive and curative medicine.

- The hot and cold theory of illness and care is influenced by the Chinese system of yin and yang and the balance between hot and cold elements. Illness, its treatment, and foods are all classified as "hot" or "cold." To cure the imbalance, foods and medicines falling under the "hot" category can be considered curative for illness caused by the "cold" group.

- Acupuncture also may be used as a way to restore the flow of energy.

Other Issues Relevant to Hospitalization   The number "4" stated in Japanese, one way, sounds like the Japanese word for "death." Providers should be aware of the implications when using this number in room assignments and teaching.

References

Easton, S. E., & Ellington, L. (1995). Japanese Americans. In A. Galens, A. Sheets, & R. V. Young (Eds), *Gale encyclopedia of multicultural America,* Vol. 2. New York: Gale Research.

Galanti, G. (1991). *Caring for patients from different cultures: Case studies for American hospitals.* Philadelphia, PA: University of Pennsylvania Press.

Ishida, D., & Inouye, J. (1995). Japanese Americans. In J. N. Giger & R. E. Davidhizar (Eds.), *Transcultural nursing: Assessment and intervention* (2nd ed.). St. Louis, MO: Mosby.

Lipson, J. G, Dibble, S. L., & Minarik, P. A. (Eds.). (1996). Japanese Americans. In *Culture and nursing care: A pocket guide.* San Francisco: University of California San Francisco Nursing Press.

Vietnam

Introduction

This information is given as an introduction to a specific culture and is meant to help providers understand similarities and variations in cultural practices. Providers are cautioned not to overgeneralize or characterize all members of a cultural or ethnic group as alike. Factors to be considered in assessing a person's cultural identity and his or her actions or beliefs include individual characteristics, socioeconomic status, race, education, religion, age, gender; the stages, conditions, and adjustment to the migration experience; and whether the family came from a rural or urban area.

This sheet is about Vietnamese traditions and practices.

Country of Origin and Geographic Location

Vietnam is a part of Southeast Asia occupying about half of the Malay Peninsula.

Language

Vietnamese is the primary language, although many Vietnamese also speak Chinese or English.

Migration Patterns

In 1975 when Communist troops invaded most of Southeast Asia, the United States government began to admit refugees from Vietnam, Cambodia, and Laos. Many Southeast Asian immigrants have experienced tremendous stress associated with their departure. They may have suffered from psychological and physical ailments as well as from the trauma of being separated from family members.

Spiritual Traditions

Many Vietnamese living in the United States practice Catholicism, although Buddhism prevails in Vietnam.

Family

The husband or eldest male is considered to be the primary decision maker in the family. In traditional Asian cultures, sons are generally given higher value than daughters.

Children are initially perceived as relatively helpless and not responsible for their actions; therefore, Southeast Asian parents always remind their children of their behavior, focusing on modeling rather than the use of strict discipline.

Mother-infant interaction is characterized by an emphasis on close physical contact. Toilet training may be introduced as early as three months of age.

Diet and Nutrition

Vietnamese who are ill may prefer to eat rice porridge sweetened with sugar.

Attitudes and General Beliefs About Illness and Death

Health care in Southeast Asia tends to be reactive, based on symptom relief. Prevention seems to be less of a priority. During the time of illness, traditional rituals and prayers are held in the home. Some may believe that illness is a punishment for faults. Traditional healing and natural medicines play an important role in health care.

Implications for Providers

Cultural Courtesies   Some of the rules regarding gestures and body language come from Buddhism.

- Vietnamese greet one another with a handshake in formal situations.

- The provider should avoid sitting or standing on a level more elevated than that of an elder. To show respect, many Southeast Asians will bow their heads to a superior or elder.

- Vietnamese tend to list their family name first, then their middle name, and their first, or given, name last.

Communication Patterns and Value Orientation   Many Vietnamese values are based on both the Confucian respect for education, family, and elders, and the Taoist desire to avoid conflict. Sparing one's feelings is considered more important than factual truth.

- To avoid confrontation or disrespect, many will not verbalize disagreement. Instead they may avoid answering a question.

- A smile should not be interpreted as happiness or agreement. Vietnamese may laugh in a situation that is, to Westerners, inappropriate. It is not necessarily a sign of ridicule or rebuke, but perhaps of nervousness.

- Speaking in a loud tone with excessive gestures is considered rude, especially when done by women.

- Summoning a person with a hand or finger in the upright position is considered derogatory. To summon a person, the entire hand with the fingers facing down is the only appropriate hand signal.

Traditional Medical Practices   Many Southeast Asian traditional medical practices are derived from Chinese medicine. This system is based on the premise that living things are composed of five basic elements: air, fire, water, earth, and metal; the associated characteristics are cold, hot, wet, and dry. One must keep all elements in proper balance to be healthy. The theory of illness is also based on the yin/yang or cold/hot classification of various diseases.

- Dermabrasive procedures based on hot/cold physiology are often used to treat coughs and other maladies.

- Cutaneous hematomas may be made over the face, neck, and trunk to release air. These are made in many different ways: by pinching and pulling on the skin, by rubbing oiled skin with the edge of a coin or spoon, or by cupping. Cupping is done by heating the air in a cup with a flame, then placing the cup on the skin.

References

Lynch, E. W., & Hanson, M. J. (Eds.). (1992). *Developing cross-cultural competence.* Baltimore, MD: Paul H. Brookes Publishing.

Office of Refugee and Immigrant Health. (1995). *Refugees and immigrants in Massachusetts: An overview of selected communities.* Boston, MA: Bureau of Family and Community Health and the Massachusetts Department of Public Health.

Chapter 3

Central America and the Caribbean

Central America and Mexico

Introduction

This information is given as an introduction to a specific culture and is meant to help providers understand similarities and variations in cultural practices. Providers are cautioned not to overgeneralize or characterize all members of a cultural or ethnic group as alike. Factors to be considered in assessing a person's cultural identity and his or her actions or beliefs include individual characteristics, socioeconomic status, race, education, religion, age, gender; the stages, conditions, and adjustment to the migration experience; and whether the family came from a rural or urban area.

This information is about families from Central America and Mexico.

Countries of Origin and Geographic Location

Belize, El Salvador, Guatemala, Costa Rica, Honduras, Nicaragua, and Panama separate the Atlantic and Pacific Ocean, on a strip of land that joins North and South America. Although Mexico is geographically a part of North America, Mexican families tend to have cultural traditions similar to those of Central Americans.

Language

Spanish is the primary and official language, although many families from Central America speak one of the many Indian dialects.

Migration Patterns

Many immigrants from Central America may have arrived as refugees, and some have been granted political asylum in the United States. Others, particularly those from Mexico, may have come to join family members here. Due to civil unrest in many Central American countries since the 1970s, there has been a rapid increase in emigration to the United States. Many immigrants may have experienced tremendous stress associated with their departure. They may have suffered from psychological and physical ailments, as well as from the trauma of being separated from family members.

Spiritual Traditions

Many Central Americans and Mexicans have roots in the Roman Catholic Church. About 25 percent belong to other Christian faiths. The Baptist church is very strong in El Salvador and Nicaragua.

Family

Single-parent families are not uncommon among these families in the United States. Women are usually responsible for the care of the children and household. Many also work night jobs. Elders often live with their children and grandchildren.

Diet and Nutrition

Rice and beans are common in the diet of Central Americans and Mexicans. Many varieties of beans (for example, garbanzos, "frijoles negros," and "gandules") are used. Other common foods include tropical fruits, root vegetables (potatoes, yucca, plantain, and ñame), tortillas, fish, and meats.

Attitudes and General Beliefs About Illness and Death

Although a public health care system exists in many Central American countries, health care is largely unavailable for people who are poor and living in rural areas. Most children in Central America have had basic immunizations but very little primary care.

Implications for Providers

Cultural Courtesies   Although many Central Americans prefer to be referred to as "Latino/a" instead of "Hispanic," it is more accurate to describe families by the country from which they come, for example, "Salvadoran" or "Guatemalan."

- Providers are generally seen as respected figures in Central American culture; however, traditional beliefs may conflict with the provider's instructions. Although the patient or family member may agree with the provider out of respect, this may not necessarily indicate that he or she intends to comply.

- Families will usually assist with most of the patient care.

- Because the extended family is the basis of these people's community, providers should discuss the care of the patient with adult family members. The father or the oldest male is often considered to be the head of the family. Medical decisions should be discussed with him, if he is present.

- Adults should be addressed by Mr. and Mrs., never by their first names, unless permission is given by the person. Women continue to use their maiden names along with their husband's family name after marriage. The last name is the mother's family name and the second to last is the father's family name. An example would be Luciana Pantos Almeidas, who would be addressed as Mrs. Pantos.

Communication Patterns and Value Orientation   It is customary to shake hands when greeting, as it is in Western culture.

- One beckons by waving all fingers with the palm down. Calling people with the palm up is considered improper.

- Pointing with the finger or hand can be misinterpreted; many finger and hand gestures are considered rude.

- Punctuality is not considered as important as it is in North America. Generally, personal relationships are more valuable. Stopping to talk to a friend or relative is more important than being on time. This is due to present-time orientation. If it is important to the provider, he or she may want to stress the importance of being on time.

Traditional Medical Practices   Some illness may be seen as resulting from supernatural or magical causes. Some adults may use traditional medicines, such as herbs or oils, to treat illness.

- A "botánica" is a store where one can buy traditional healing herbs and oils.

- Healers, often called "curandero," "sobador," or "horchún," use traditional healing methods.

Other Issues Relevant to Hospitalization   Many recent immigrants have no more than a middle school education, while others are trained and educated professionals. The provider may want to provide education verbally and visually, as well as in writing.

References

Council of Churches of Greater Springfield and the Visiting Nurse Hospice of Pioneer Valley. (1995). *Knowing my neighbor: Religious beliefs and cultural traditions at times of illness and death.* Springfield, MA: Council of Churches.

David Kennedy Center for International Studies. (1996). *Culturgrams: El Salvador, Guatemala, Honduras, Mexico.* Provo, UT: Brigham Young University.

Lynch, E. W., & Hanson, M. J. (Eds.). (1992). *Developing cross-cultural competencies.* Baltimore, MD: Paul H. Brookes Publishing.

Office of Refugee and Immigrant Health. (1995). *Refugees and immigrants in Massachusetts: An overview of selected communities.* Boston, MA: Bureau of Family and Community Health and the Massachusetts Department of Public Health.

Samolsky, S., Dunker, K., & Hynak-Hankinson, M. T . (1990). Feeding the Hispanic hospital patient: Cultural considerations. *Journal of the American Dietetic Association, 90* (12), 1707–1710.

Spector, R. (1996). *Cultural diversity in health and illness* (4th ed.). Stamford, CT: Appleton & Lange.

Websites: *www.texmed.org* and *www2.epixnet/~escobar/vista.html*

Dominican Republic

Introduction

This information is given as an introduction to a specific culture and is meant to help providers understand similarities and variations in cultural practices. Providers are cautioned not to overgeneralize or characterize all members of a cultural or ethnic group as alike. Factors to be considered in assessing a person's cultural identity and his or her actions or beliefs include individual characteristics, socioeconomic status, race, education, religion, age, gender; the stages, conditions, and adjustment to the migration experience; and whether the family came from a rural or urban area.

The following information is provided about traditions and practices in the Dominican Republic.

Country of Origin and Geographic Location

The Dominican Republic is located in the Caribbean Sea. It shares the island of Hispaniola with Haiti.

Language

Spanish is spoken.

Migration Patterns

Dominicans have been immigrating to the United States since the 1960s. During the 1980s, the Dominican Republic became the sixth largest source of legal immigration to the United States.

Spiritual Traditions

The majority of Dominicans are Roman Catholic.

Family

As in other Latino cultures, the immediate and extended family is the center of social activities, major decision making, and daily life. The father may be the primary decision maker, whereas the mother may provide the majority of care.

Diet and Nutrition

The Dominican diet consists of foods with their origins in Indian, Spanish, and African cultures. Rice and beans are common. Many varieties of beans (for example, garbanzos, "frijoles negros," and "gandules") are used. Other common foods include tropical fruits, root vegetables (potatoes, yucca, plantain, and ñame are examples), fish, and meats.

Attitudes and General Beliefs About Illness and Death

Dominicans tend to live in close-knit communities; therefore, many cultural values and health traditions remain strong. Extended families are sources of support for the ill. Customs and rituals surrounding death are often aligned with the Roman Catholic faith.

Implications for Providers

Cultural Courtesies   Although many people of Latin-American descent prefer to be referred to as "Latino" rather than "Hispanic," it is more accurate to describe families by the country from which they come, for example, "Dominican."

- Providers are generally seen as respected figures in Dominican culture; however, traditional beliefs may conflict with the instructions of the provider. Although the patient or family member may agree with the provider out of respect, this may not necessarily indicate that he or she intends to comply.

- Families will usually assist with most of the patient care. Because the extended family is the basis of their community, providers should discuss the care of the patient with the adult family members.

- The father or the oldest male is often considered to be the head of the family. Medical decisions should be discussed with him, if he is present; however, it is most often that the mother or grandmother will carry out the medical instructions.

Communication Patterns and Value Orientation   It is customary to shake hands when greeting.

- Dominicans may stand in close groups. When they are talking, they may gesture with their hands.

- During a conversation, members of a group may interrupt one another. This would not be considered rude.

- In Latino culture, taking time to nurture personal relationships is considered more important than being on time. One may risk being late for an appointment to stop and talk with a friend. As with all families, the provider may want to explain the importance of being on time for appointments.

Traditional Medical Practices   Many traditional practices come from the Caribbean's African influence.

- An "espiritista" is a person who is believed to have spiritual powers for curing diseases and controlling spirits.

- A "botánica" is a resource store in the Latino community where families can buy herbs and other more traditional remedies.

- Some Dominican families may refer to the espiritista or botánica before going to the physician or clinic.

References

Council of Churches of Greater Springfield and the Visiting Nurse Hospice of Pioneer Valley. (1995). *Knowing my neighbor: Religious beliefs and cultural traditions at times of illness and death.* Springfield, MA: Council of Churches.

Garcia-Preto, N. (1996). Latino families. In M. McGoldrick, J. Giordano, & J. K. Pearce (Eds.), *Ethnicity and family therapy* (2nd ed.). New York: Guilford Press.

Lynch, E. W., & Hanson, M. J. (Eds). (1992). *Developing cross-cultural competencies.* Baltimore, MD: Paul H. Brookes Publishing.

Haiti

Introduction

This information is given as an introduction to a specific culture and is meant to help providers understand similarities and variations in cultural practices. Providers are cautioned not to overgeneralize or characterize all members of a cultural or ethnic group as alike. Factors to be considered in assessing a person's cultural identity and his or her actions or beliefs include individual characteristics, socioeconomic status, race, education, religion, age, gender; the stages, conditions, and adjustment to the migration experience; and whether the family came from a rural or urban area.

This information is about Haitian traditions and practices.

Country of Origin and Geographic Location

Haiti is located in the Caribbean Sea. It shares the island of Hispaniola with the Dominican Republic.

Language

The primary language is Creole (Kreol). Although French is the official language of Haiti, only 2 to 5 percent of the Haitian population speaks French fluently.

Migration Patterns

Many Haitians have left the country to escape poverty and political turmoil. Most Haitian migratory experiences include the disruption of social and psychological support systems.

Spiritual Traditions

Religion is a dominant force in the Haitian community. Although the government-sanctioned religion is Roman Catholicism, Vodoun ("voodoo") is practiced widely. Over the last four decades there has been a growing influence of various Protestant groups, as well, including evangelical movements in both Haiti and the United States.

Family

Many Haitian couples are married by common law. Husbands are expected to be financial providers and child disciplinarians, while daily child-rearing responsibilities are delegated to women. Many grandparents live in the home and provide care of the grandchildren while parents are at work. In many Haitian families, parent-child roles tend to be clearly delineated, with limited tolerance for the child's self-expression. Children often learn not to ask questions, as conformity and obedience are expected. It is important for the provider to consider the opinions and ideas of extended family members in planning the patient's medical care.

Diet and Nutrition

Haitian food tends to be spicy, and most dishes are cooked in oil. Many women will avoid certain foods during pregnancy, after delivery, and at certain times of the month.

Attitudes and General Beliefs About Illness and Death

Although a public health care system exists in Haiti, it is largely unavailable for people who are poor and those in remote areas. Most children in Haiti have had basic immunizations but very little primary care.

Implications for Providers

Cultural Courtesies   Most Haitians say that they find touch from providers to be supportive, comforting, and reassuring. Avoidance of direct eye contact is considered to be a sign of respect.

Communication Patterns and Value Orientation   Many Haitians, like most families with few financial resources, tend to live in the present moment. They may view future-oriented tasks as unimportant or less relevant than the present.

- Inability to keep appointments and the discontinuation of medication after disappearance of symptoms may be related to present-time orientation and lack of knowledge about preventive care.

- Most immigrants from Haiti have great admiration for nurses; nurses are often given more respect than physicians in Haiti.

Traditional Medical Practices   The practice of Vodoun ("voodoo") is founded in the belief that people are surrounded by powerful spirits. It is believed that it is necessary to invoke spirits to cure illness.

- Haitians may go to a Vodoun priest for healing.
- In the Haitian culture, the spirits are called "loas," "mysteres," or "saints."

- A Vodoun priest is known as a "shaman" (Vodoun practitioner), herbalist or "docte fey," midwife, bonesetter or "docté zo," or "injectionist pikirist."
- Bottle-feeding is considered unnatural by many Haitian women.

Other Issues Relevant to Hospitalization   During the 1980s, Haiti was rumored to be a possible source from which AIDS was imported into the United States. In some instances, AIDS became known as a "Haitian disease." This theory has long since been abandoned; however, for many people, the stigma remains. This experience of stigmatization may affect the Haitian family's trust (or lack thereof) for the health care provider.

- Major factors contributing to the incidence of diarrhea and dehydration among newborns of recent immigrants are the cultural beliefs surrounding newborn nourishment and purging. For many Haitians, diarrhea may signify a cleansing of the body that is essential for health maintenance and illness prevention or cure. They may not feed a baby who has diarrhea.

- Proper respect for traditional health beliefs will help to gain the family's respect and cooperation. Rejection of a family's cultural beliefs may result in mistrust of the health provider as well as the plan of care.

References

Bibb, A., & Casimir, G. (1996). Haitian families. In M. McGoldrick, J. Giordano, & J. Pearce. (Eds.), *Ethnicity and family therapy* (2nd ed.). New York: Guilford Press.

Colin, J. M., & Paperwala, G. (1996). Haitians. In J. G. Lipson, S. L. Dibble, & P. A. Minarik (Eds.), *Culture and care: A pocket guide.* San Francisco: University of California San Francisco Nursing Press.

DeSantis, L. (1988). Cultural factors affecting newborn and infant diarrhea. *Journal of Pediatric Nursing, 3*(6), 391–398.

Giger, J. N., & Davidhizar, R. E. (1995). *Transcultural nursing: Assessment and intervention* (2nd ed.). St. Louis, MO: Mosby.

Giger, J., Davidhizar, R., Parsons, L., & Holcomb, L. (1996). Haitian Americans: Implications for nursing care. *Journal of Community Health Nursing, 13*(4), 249–260.

Website: *www.geocities.com/athens/Delphi/5319*

Chapter 4

Europe

Greece

Introduction

This information is given as an introduction to a specific culture and is meant to help providers understand similarities and variations in cultural practices. Providers are cautioned not to overgeneralize or characterize all members of a cultural or ethnic group as alike. Factors to be considered in assessing a person's cultural identity and his or her actions or beliefs include individual characteristics, socioeconomic status, race, education, religion, age, gender; the stages, conditions, and adjustment to the migration experience; and whether the family came from a rural or urban area.

The following information is about Greek traditions and practices.

Country of Origin and Geographic Location

Greece is located in Eastern Europe between the Mediterranean and Aegean Seas.

Language

Greek is the language of the country.

Migration Patterns

Many Greeks have come to this country seeking better economic conditions. Many have also come to the United States for educational opportunities.

Spiritual Traditions

Approximately 98 percent of the Greek population practices the Eastern Orthodox religion. The church in Greece is very important to the social and community structure.

Family

The extended family is very important in Greek culture. Individual needs are generally seen as less important than family needs. If a mother works, the grandmother will probably play a major role in the rearing of the children and often will be influential regarding the care of a child.

Diet and Nutrition

Many Greeks do not eat meat on Wednesday or Friday. During Holy Week before the Greek Orthodox Easter (usually in April), Greeks may abstain from all dairy products, meat, fish, and olive oil. This tradition is usually waived for a patient.

Attitudes and General Beliefs About Illness and Death

Many people of Greek origin derive strength from their religion. During illness, they may ask for a Greek priest to visit them or may want to go to a Greek Orthodox church to pray and light candles. It is common for parents to ask if an icon, cross, or other religious item may be brought into the operating room during surgery for protection of their child.

Implications for Providers

Cultural Courtesies   It is customary to shake hands when greeting, as in other Western cultures.

- It is considered courteous for providers to learn to pronounce the child's Greek name, rather than to shorten it.

- Elders in the family are respected and are addressed as Mr. or Mrs.

- Sharing or offering food is seen as an important gesture of hospitality.

- Family members may make meals for patients. Any restrictions should be clarified with family or visitors.

- The father or the oldest male is often considered to be the head of the family. Medical care should be discussed with him, if he is present.

Communication Patterns and Value Orientation   Tilting one's head upward as a reaction to a statement or a question means "no"; the sound "tssk" represents an emphatic "no."

- The provider's facial expressions may be read for signs of how the child is doing.

- A positive expression, such as a smile, is interpreted as encouraging.

Traditional Medical Practices   Many Greeks believe that one can prevent illness with proper exercise and a healthy diet of Greek foods. A charm (usually a blue bead) is often believed to protect one from negative forces.

Other Issues Relevant to Hospitalization

There are no other general issues related to hospitalization of members of the Greek culture.

References

Council of Churches of Greater Springfield and the Visiting Nurse Hospice of Pioneer Valley. (1995). *Knowing my neighbor: Religious beliefs and cultural traditions at times of illness and death.* Springfield, MA: Council of Churches.

Leininger, M. (Ed.). (1991). *Culture care diversity and universality: A theory of nursing.* New York: National League of Nursing.

Tsemberis, S. J. (1996). Greek families. In M. McGoldrick, J. Giordano, & J. K. Pearce (Eds.), *Ethnicity and family therapy* (2nd ed.). New York: Guilford Press.

Gypsies (Roma)

Introduction

This information is given as an introduction to a specific culture and is meant to help providers understand similarities and variations in cultural practices. Providers are cautioned not to overgeneralize or characterize all members of a cultural or ethnic group as alike. Factors to be considered in assessing a person's cultural identity and his or her actions or beliefs include individual characteristics, socioeconomic status, race, education, religion, age, gender; the stages, conditions, and adjustment to the migration experience; and whether the family came from a rural or urban area.

The following information is about Gypsy or Roma traditions and practices.

Country of Origin and Geographic Location

The Gypsy culture is known as Roma, Rom, or Romani, as well as other names. Most Gypsy families identify themselves by a name with the prefix "Rom." While most understand and use the term "Gypsy," it is seen as derogatory. In this book, the term "Roma" will be used to describe the Gypsy population.

Roma most likely originated in India around 1,000 A.D. The Roma have since traveled and settled in many different European countries. The population has experienced many divisions and separations. This has made it difficult to place the Roma into one ethnic category. There are approximately twelve million Roma living in the world today.

Language

There are many spoken dialects of the Roma language. Those from Western Europe and the majority in the United States speak Romany (also known as Romanes or Romani). Because many dialects are not written, history has been maintained through an oral tradition of storytelling. All of the dialects are based on Punjabi or Hindi but have traces of other languages in them (most likely influences from the many countries in which Roma have lived). A family may also speak the language of the country of origin.

Migration Patterns

Roma families have settled throughout the United States. Those currently living in the United States were most likely born here, and many have adapted to many of the social and cultural norms of U.S. society. Most live a less nomadic lifestyle, no longer moving from campground to campground. This is antithetical to Roma lifestyle, which holds that isolation away from dominant society is crucial to the integrity of the culture.

Spiritual Traditions

Some Roma practice the religions of their homelands, such as Christianity or Islam. Yet most practice a religion similar to Wicca, believing in the existence of God and Satan, good and bad luck, and the supernatural.

Family

Family in Roma culture consists of extended family members who may not necessarily be related by blood. It is a strong, tight unit, known as a clan or "kumpania." The clan often lives together, works together, and shares major events. The elder members of each clan are considered to be the authority figures and decision makers in all cases. In a health care setting, providers should speak to the elders when decisions must be made.

Many Roma children never enter the public school system. If they do, they enroll late or are removed early. This is to ensure as little contact as possible with the non-Roma ("Gadje") world. This, combined with a high rate of illiteracy, ensures little knowledge of the English language or of current events.

Diet and Nutrition

The strong cultural beliefs about purity and cleanliness create a source of conflict in a hospital, where the source of food is unknown to Roma visitors. They do not want any contact with the non-Roma world, and therefore avoid hospital food, plates, and trays. Older Roma may want to eat their own food, such as packaged, canned, or pre-wrapped items. Younger children may not acknowledge the culture's strict dietary rules, so they can usually eat hospital food that is given to them. Allow the patient or family to remove the plastic cover from utensils and dishes that arrive from the hospital cafeteria. Provide sterile, plastic, disposable utensils whenever possible.

The dietary trends of the Roma in the United States have led to growing health problems. Their diet may consist of high levels of fat and cholesterol and may lack necessary nutrients. This may be the result of a lack of financial resources or little knowledge about healthy food choices. Roma also believe that being heavy or fat symbolizes health and good fortune, while being thin is associated with poverty and illness. They will therefore not be inclined to lose weight or be knowledgeable about illness associated with obesity.

Attitudes and General Beliefs About Illness and Death

The most important cultural belief of the Roma community is that of purity and cleanliness. Purity is maintained by avoiding Gadje and not entering the Gadje world. They consider their world clean as long as there is no contamination from the Western world. Cross-contamination is thought to cause pollution ("marimé"), which could bring illness or even death. The hospital, therefore, is not an easy place for a Roma family to come, being filled with the pollutants of the non-Roma society. Hospitalization is generally a last resort, as the stress that it causes in the Roma community can be as great as the illness itself.

Individual purity is maintained by separating the upper half of the body (considered "clean") from the lower half of the body (considered "unclean"). Extra towels and soaps will be needed in order to maintain this cleanliness. Washing is done in running water. Roma only take showers; no baths are taken. Clothes of women and men are not washed together.

Women who are menstruating or pregnant are considered contaminated; they must wash their clothes and bathe away from the other members of the family. Women are not allowed to cook during menstruation.

Postpartum women are considered contaminated for nine days following birth. During this time they must not touch men. Older women from the community will tend to surround the new mother, while immediate family members may not be present.

The cause of illness among Roma is believed to be pollution. Pollution comes from non-Roma interaction, and illness can also come from not following the traditional Roma rules regarding purity. Illness can also be caused by committing a sin or by ghosts or spirits invading the body. Roma families may turn to Western or non-Roma medicine if absolutely necessary. For example, if the illness is believed to be caused by non-Roma pollution, they will go to a Western provider.

If a Western doctor is known to have cured a Roma, the Roma community will soon know about it. Because trust is a major aspect of health care, the doctor who has developed a successful relationship with one Roma family may soon begin to see others.

The death of a Roma, and subsequent funeral, is a major community event. Roma communities will travel great distances to be with the grieving family or to attend the funeral. In a case in which a baby dies, the parents may avoid the deceased and may even leave the hospital. They leave the burial arrangements to other community members, who may also leave to avoid bad luck associated with death. Grieving behaviors include moaning, scratching one's face, or pulling one's hair.

Implications for Providers

Cultural Courtesies   Roma focus on "big" names and status positions. For example, the family may wish to see the "head doctor" in a certain department or the most well-known name in a particular specialty. This may have something to do with the provider's past performance or "cure rate," that is, how many other Roma have developed a relationship with the provider.

- Roma greet one another by waving with the palm up.

- Roma family names may be confusing to doctors and nurses. One Roma family may have many different last names. Names may have more to do with the clan or country of origin than the husband or father's surname. Therefore, an immediate family member or very close relative may appear unrelated. First names may be used to address people, as opposed to the use of the surname.

- Because Roma consider areas below the waist to be unclean, body fluids such as urine or bowel movements, and the discussion of them, are sensitive issues. This is especially true for women during menstruation or after childbirth.

- Examinations by a male physician may be uncomfortable for the female patient. The provider should be clear about the need for such an examination, as it may be considered shameful.

- Modesty is very important to Roma women. They may prefer to wear their own clothing instead of hospital garments.

Communication Patterns and Value Orientation   Communication among group members may appear aggressive and argumentative by North American standards.

- Shouting does not necessarily mean that Roma are arguing or disagree with one another.

- Communication with a Roma family starts with the elder members. They can then relay the important news to the younger members.

Traditional Medical Practices   When a Roma is near death or deceased, the family and Roma community may gather around the patient.

They ask for forgiveness of bad deeds done to that person, so that the deceased will not come back as an evil spirit.

- Some Roma communities plug the deceased's nostrils so that evil spirits cannot enter the body.

- Some women in the Roma community, known as "drabarni" or "drabegni," practice traditional medicine.

Other Issues Relevant to Hospitalization

Although younger members of the family may be the most likely to speak and read English, they should not be used to interpret for the family.

- The entire Roma community often joins the immediate family in support of the patient. The patient will not be left alone. Often visiting rules are broken so that someone can always stay with the patient. The noisier and less private the hospital room, the better.

- Frequent washing of hands is also vital to fight pollution or contamination.

References

Dean, J. M., Rogers, M. C., & Wetzel, R. C. (1983, November). The art of pediatrics: Gypsies and acute medical intervention. *Pediatrics, 72*(5), 731–735.

Fonseca, I. Among the Gypsies. (1995, September 25). *The New Yorker*, pp. 84–97.

Ghada, K. (1993). *The ethnic handbook.* Cambridge, MA: Blackwell Science.

Häggblom, M., Heldt, H., Horte, A., Hähkönen, J., Kero, J., Möttönen, M., Ojanlatva, A., Saraste, A., Turunen, T., & Vandenbussche, C. (1997). The use of problem-based learning in dealing with cultural minority groups. *Patient Education and Counseling, 31,* 171–176.

Mandell, F. (1974). Gypsies: Culture and child care. *Pediatrics, 54*(5), 603–607.

McKee, M. (1997, November 8). The health of Gypsies. *British Medical Journal, 315,* 1172–1173.

Sutherland, A. H. (1997). Gypsies. In J. G. Lipson, S. L. Dibble, & P. A. Minarik (Eds.). (1997). *Culture and nursing care: A pocket guide.* San Francisco: University of California San Francisco Nursing Press.

Websites: *www.religious tolerance.org.* and *www.romani.org*

Portugal

Introduction

This information is given as an introduction to a specific culture and is meant to help providers understand similarities and variations in cultural practices. Providers are cautioned not to overgeneralize or characterize all members of a cultural or ethnic group as alike. Factors to be considered in assessing a person's cultural identity and his or her actions or beliefs include individual characteristics, socioeconomic status, race, education, religion, age, gender; the stages, conditions, and adjustment to the migration experience; and whether the family came from a rural or urban area.

The following information is about Portuguese traditions and practices.

Country of Origin and Geographic Location

Continental Portugal is in Western Europe on the Iberian Peninsula, which it shares with Spain. The archipelagos of Azores and Madeira, also part of Portugal, are in the Atlantic Ocean.

Language

Portuguese is the official language of Portugal.

Migration Patterns

Of the 1.5 million people of Portuguese origin living in the United States, most have settled in the New England states, New Jersey, California, and Hawaii. There have been several stages of immigration during the last century. Different groups have different job skills and education levels.

Some Portuguese have migrated to and from other countries, including Brazil or Portugal's former colonies of Angola, Mozambique, Guinea Bissau, or Cape Verde.

Spiritual Traditions

Approximately 97 percent of the Portuguese population is Catholic. Some Portuguese have converted to evangelical religions.

Family

Portuguese families are traditionally patriarchal (the father is the decision maker); however, many families have allowed for more shared responsibility within the family. In Portuguese culture, mothers are generally in charge of the household. Extended families are a strong source of emotional and financial support. Godparents and elders are very important and highly respected members of the family. Children are a source of great happiness and are the center of attention; however, they are expected to be seen and not heard. Discipline in Portuguese families includes shame and guilt-inducing techniques. Spanking is common, but there is a clear distinction between discipline and abusive punishment.

Diet and Nutrition

The staple foods in Portugal are fish, chicken, and a variety of meats that are cooked in many ways. Dishes are often seasoned with tomatoes and onions and garlic. Food is usually cooked in olive oil. Fruits and vegetables are important in the diet. Wine, which is served with meals, is seen as having special benefits for the blood.

Attitudes and General Beliefs About Illness and Death

Religion and prayer are very important when coping with illness. Some Portuguese may say prayers and make promises to saints, especially to Our Lady of Fatima and Santo Cristo. Portuguese tend to view illness as an event out of their control or governed by fate. Some may believe in the "evil eye" and illness as a punishment for wrongdoing. Among family and trusted friends, illness is often discussed and analyzed; however, they may avoid asking important questions of the provider for fear of the worst possible news.

Implications for Providers

Cultural Courtesies   Most Portuguese can be described as reserved, traditional, and conservative. The health care provider might consider this when communicating with the family and take time to develop the relationship. Have the patient and family understand the importance of sharing thoughts and feelings in implementing the treatment plan.

Communication Patterns and Value Orientation   Probing questions may be startling and met with resistance, as Portuguese tend to be reserved.

- Women in the family will be very helpful in making decisions, and they will know how to approach the father or the husband. The provider might want to approach the woman or the mother first.
- Araujo (1996, p. 588) writes that key values to the Portuguese culture are "honra" (honor), "respeito" (respect), "bondade" (goodness), and "confianca" (trust).

- Showing respect toward the provider means they may agree with the care plan when they really do not. When a good rapport with the provider has been established, the family will trust him or her more and be open to discussing the illness and treatment. Providers are advised to discuss the illness with tact and allow the family to approach it in their own way.

- The concept of "goodness" means that they will think of others before themselves. Portuguese may be reluctant to ask for help for fear of imposing, yet they assume that help will be offered or needs will be met when the patient or family is experiencing difficulties.

Traditional Medical Practices   To supplement Western medical care, Portuguese may seek the help of a "curandeiro," who is thought to have supernatural powers for healing. The curandeiro may use prayer or herbs or oils to help with the healing. An "endireita" (lay osteopath) may be sought for problems related to bones.

- Herbal teas are often used for certain ailments.

- Illness may be attributed to getting cold or "catching a draft."

Other Issues Relevant to Hospitalization   Faith in God is strong among Portuguese immigrants and would probably override the desire to seek extraordinary means in keeping a patient alive.

- Believers in the evil eye may wear amulets or have someone pray for them or their home.

- Some patients may not understand the need for frequent blood tests. The provider should explain the process of blood regeneration if necessary.

References

Araujo, Z. (1996). Portuguese families. In M. McGoldrick, J. Giordano, & J. K. Pearce (Eds.), *Ethnicity and family therapy* (2nd ed.). New York: Guilford Press.

Council of Churches of Greater Springfield and the Visiting Nurse Hospice of Pioneer Valley. (1995). *Knowing my neighbor: Religious beliefs and cultural traditions at times of illness and death.* Springfield, MA: Council of Churches.

Office of Refugee and Immigrant Health. (1995). *Refugees and immigrants in Massachusetts: An overview of selected communities.* Boston, MA: Bureau of Family and Community Health and the Massachusetts Department of Public Health.

Russia

Introduction

This information is given as an introduction to a specific culture and is meant to help providers understand similarities and variations in cultural practices. Providers are cautioned not to overgeneralize or characterize all members of a cultural or ethnic group as alike. Factors to be considered in assessing a person's cultural identity and his or her actions or beliefs include individual characteristics, socioeconomic status, race, education, religion, age, gender; the stages, conditions, and adjustment to the migration experience; and whether the family came from a rural or urban area.

The following information is about Russian traditions and practices.

Country of Origin and Geographic Location

Russia was a state of the former Soviet Union in Eastern Europe.

Language

Russian is spoken.

Migration Patterns

Emigration from Russia was banned for all but a few until 1991. The current wave of Russian immigrants largely consists of members of the educated, professional class.

Spiritual Traditions

During the Communist era, religious services were prohibited and often brought dire consequences, particularly among Jews. The majority of Russian immigrants are Jewish, nonpracticing or atheist, and Muslim.

Family

In Russia, children represent the family's hope for the future; they are seen as symbols of innocence and are often overprotected. One-child families predominate; extended family members are close and often become substitute brothers and sisters. Women traditionally raise the family, and grandmothers are usually involved in child care. In Russia, parents rely on the school system to provide structure and limits.

Diet and Nutrition

The Russian diet reflects the scarcity of fresh food in the region. Staples are boiled meats, pickled vegetables, and potatoes.

Attitudes and General Beliefs About Illness and Death

The focus of medicine in Russia is on revealing the cause of the illness. Doctors in Russia are judged by their ability to find the cause and treat the illness. A doctor who does not have an immediate solution to a problem may not be as well-respected.

In Russia, families are assigned to a particular physician. Whether or not they trust their health care provider depends largely on his or her personality, concern, professionalism, and awareness of the differences among health care services.

Suffering is often seen as having redemptive value. Pain and misfortune are accepted, yet dealt with privately. Parents and patients might be reluctant to discuss emotional suffering with outsiders.

Historically, emotional and mental health problems were not discussed, even among family members. Russians in the United States may need to be made aware of the mental health benefits available to them.

Implications for Providers

Cultural Courtesies   Russian families may prefer to remain at a social distance, rather than at an intimate distance with health care providers. If this social distance must be breached in order to provide care, a careful explanation should be given first.

- Touch is often used freely among Russians with intimate and close friends.

- Eye contact is freely used as a sign of respect and trust.

- Health care providers should address parents using the family's last name. Many Russians object to the use of terms of endearment, such as "honey."

Communication Patterns and Value Orientation   Many Russian parents are used to fighting for their child's rights, and they may insist on having their child stay longer or ask for more diagnostic services. Assuring the parent that the provider's primary concern is the child's welfare may ease any worries.

- Russians expect formality in the health care setting. They tend not to appreciate a lighthearted or "chatty" approach to health care.

- As non-native English speakers, Russians expect providers to use simple words. Because many Russians are highly educated, they may hesitate to say that they do not understand something. Asking parents or patients to repeat back what was said to them will give a provider a better idea of their understanding.

Traditional Medical Practices   Traditional remedies are used in Russia, along with conventional medicine. Traditional remedies are considered by many Russians to be less harmful than chemical medicine and may include herbs, massage, and dry heat.

- A common medication is "zelenka," a mercurochrome-based green ointment for skin problems.

- Asking parents what they have tried at home or what was helpful in the past may be important for patient and parent compliance with the provider's recommendations.

- In Russia, psychiatric illness was often treated with strong sedatives and institutionalization. Russian immigrants may be very skeptical of mental health services.

Other Issues Relevant to Hospitalization   In Russia, universal health care is provided for everyone in the country. There are, however, no primary care providers, and patients do not choose their own doctors.

- Russians may be accustomed to longer lengths of stay than are typical in the United States. In Russia, newborns stay in the hospital for one week after a normal birth, and the average in-patient stay is three weeks.

- Helping patients and parents understand the differences between the Russian and the U.S. health care systems and how to navigate the U.S. health care system are important components of care.

References

Althausen, L. (1996). Russian families. In M. McGoldrick, J. Giordano, & J. K. Pearce (Eds.), *Ethnicity and family therapy* (2nd ed.). New York: Guilford Press.

Elyasberg, Y. (1996). Voices of the Soviet Jewish community. University of Washington, Healthlinks. Ethnomed: *www.hslib.washington.edu/clinical/ethnomed/voices/sovjew.html*

Giger, J. N., & Davidhizar, R. E. (1995). *Transcultural nursing: Assessment and intervention* (2nd ed.). St. Louis, MO: Mosby.

Chapter 5

The Middle East

Saudi Arabia

Introduction

This information is given as an introduction to a specific culture and is meant to help providers understand similarities and variations in cultural practices. Providers are cautioned not to overgeneralize or characterize all members of a cultural or ethnic group as alike. Factors to be considered in assessing a person's cultural identity and his or her actions or beliefs include individual characteristics, socioeconomic status, race, education, religion, age, gender; the stages, conditions, and adjustment to the migration experience; and whether the family came from a rural or urban area.

The following information is about Saudi traditions and practices.

Country of Origin and Geographic Location

The Kingdom of Saudi Arabia sits on the Arabian Peninsula, bordered by the Red Sea and the Persian Gulf.

Language

Arabic is the official language of the kingdom. Many Saudis speak fluent English, which is used in business and educational settings.

Migration Patterns

Many Saudis come to the United States temporarily for business or educational purposes.

Spiritual Traditions

Islam (the faith of Muslims) is the only legally and officially recognized religion of Saudi Arabia, although some Saudis living in the United States may practice Christianity. The Arabian Peninsula is the center of the Islamic religion, which has spread throughout the world.

Family

Family honor is very important to Saudi culture. In all matters, one is expected to place family or group concerns before any individual concerns. Families are generally patriarchal. Fathers are the primary decision makers, yet women may exercise considerable influence in the home.

Diet and Nutrition

Saudi dishes include rice with lamb or chicken and are mildly spicy. Coffee or tea is served before all meals. Buttermilk and camel's milk are popular drinks. Muslims do not eat pork or drink alcohol. Those who are Muslim may prefer to eat "halal" meat. Halal (that which is permissible by Islamic law) refers to the method of preparation for consumption. If halal meat is not available, many will accept kosher meat as a substitute.

Attitudes and General Beliefs About Illness and Death

Many general Saudi beliefs stem from the Muslim tradition. Religious teachings give meaning to aspects of life, death, child rearing, and the maintenance and cause of illness. In Saudi Arabia, medical care is free. Many who come to the United States for medical care are subsidized by the Saudi Embassy.

Implications for Providers

Cultural Courtesies   Males and females are generally separated in Saudi social and business circles. Rules governing the actions of Saudi women are based on Saudi law and custom and are designed to protect a woman's modesty and honor.

- It is impolite to point with a finger or signal to another person with the hand, especially the left hand.

- It is also considered an insult to point the bottom of one's foot at another person or to cross the ankle over the knee.

- In Saudi Arabia, female doctors treat women and children.

Communication Patterns and Value Orientation   In accordance with the teachings of Islam, which espouse modesty, it is proper for one to lower the gaze and avoid direct eye contact when meeting someone of the opposite sex.

- When greeting, it is considered proper to shake hands with the right hand.

- When accompanied by a woman wearing a veil, a man will not normally introduce her, and one does not expect to shake hands with her.

Other Issues Relevant to Hospitalization   Many Muslim women do not expose any skin, except for their hands and part of their face, to any man except for their husband or child. Providers are advised to put signs on patient rooms to knock before entering, so that the woman might cover herself before meeting guests.

References

David Kennedy Center for International Studies. (1996). *Culturgrams: Saudi Arabia.* Provo, UT: Brigham Young University.

Luna, L. J. (1989, Summer). Transcultural nursing care of Arab Muslims. *Journal of Transcultural Nursing, 1*(1), 22–26.

Chapter 6

South America

Brazil

Introduction

This information is given as an introduction to a specific culture and is meant to help providers understand similarities and variations in cultural practices. Providers are cautioned not to overgeneralize or characterize all members of a cultural or ethnic group as alike. Factors to be considered in assessing a person's cultural identity and his or her actions or beliefs include individual characteristics, socioeconomic status, race, education, religion, age, gender; the stages, conditions, and adjustment to the migration experience; and whether the family came from a rural or urban area.

The following information is about Brazilian traditions and practices.

Country of Origin and Geographic Location

Brazil is located in South America, the bulk between the equator and the Tropic of Capricorn.

Language

Portuguese is the official language.

Migration Patterns

Brazilian immigrants in the United States say that they have come to the United States due to unstable economic conditions in Brazil. Many professionals come to the United States to pursue education, as well as business and professional goals. Large Brazilian communities exist in California, Florida, and New York.

Spiritual Traditions

Catholicism is the dominant religion in Brazil. The Evangelical Christian Protestant, Jewish, and Esperitism communities are growing. The African religions "Condomble" and "Umbanda" play a part in many Catholic communities, as does Liberation Theology.

Family

Brazilian family structure includes not only immediate members, but also extended family and close friends. All involve themselves in family conflicts and their resolution (Korin, 1996).

Grandparents and godparents may be involved in decision making concerning health care. Loyalty to the family is an important value in the Brazilian culture.

Diet and Nutrition

Two popular dishes are "feijoada" (black beans with beef, pork, and sausage) and "churrasco," a variety of grilled meats. Many dishes are served with beans, rice, greens, salad, and root vegetables. Tropical fruits and fruit juices are popular.

Attitudes and General Beliefs About Illness and Death

In Brazil, public and private health institutions are quite separate. Excellent medical care is available in big cities for those who can afford private care. However, other, more remote areas only have access to public facilities, which are often ill equipped. Those using private health care facilities are more affluent, perhaps have received more education, and have higher expectations of treatment. Brazilians may hesitate to question medical authority.

Implications for Providers

Cultural Courtesies   Warmth and respect are important in relationships. "Brazilians respond better to a friendly, personal manner rather than a businesslike one, expecting the care provider to be personally interested in their problems and to take an active role in their lives" (Korin, 1996, p. 207). This is especially true regarding children's issues.

Communication Patterns and Value Orientation   Expressions of grief may be very intense and demonstrative.

Brazilian culture has roots in both Portugal and Africa. Race relations and identification are more complex and have different connotations than in the United States.

Traditional Medical Practices   Alternative medicine (herbs and spiritual approaches) may be used among certain subgroups.

Other Issues Relevant to Hospitalization   Autopsies might be viewed negatively. New ideas are emerging related to the importance of organ donation and transplantation.

In Brazil, funerals take place within twenty-four hours of death. Families will follow American burial customs when in the United States.

References

David Kennedy Center for International Studies. (1997). *Culturgrams: Brazil.* Provo, UT: Brigham Young University.

Korin, E. K. (1996). Brazilian families. In M. McGoldrick, J. Giordano, & J. K. Pearce (Eds.), *Ethnicity and family therapy* (2nd ed.). New York: Guilford Press.

Office of Refugee and Immigrant Health. (1995). *Refugees and immigrants in Massachusetts: An overview of selected communities.* Boston, MA: Bureau of Family and Community Health and the Massachusetts Department of Public Health.

Chapter 7

North America

African American

Introduction

This information is given as an introduction to a specific culture and is meant to help providers understand similarities and variations in cultural practices. Providers are cautioned not to overgeneralize or characterize all members of a cultural or ethnic group as alike. Factors to be considered in assessing a person's cultural identity and his or her actions or beliefs include individual characteristics, socioeconomic status, race, education, religion, age, gender; the stages, conditions, and adjustment to the migration experience; and whether the family came from a rural or urban area.

The following information is about African American traditions.

Country of Origin and Geographic Location

African Americans constitute about 12 percent of the U.S. population. The African American population includes descendants of slaves brought to this country from 1518 to 1870, immigrants from the Caribbean, and more recent immigrants from many countries in Africa. This information focuses primarily on African Americans whose families have lived in the United States for up to three hundred years.

Language

Although African Americans speak English, those from the rural South may have distinct accents and use terms unfamiliar to those from the north. In addition, some may use a distinct style of speech generally termed "ebonics." It is important to note that although some African Americans may use different speech patterns, this should not be mistaken for lack of intelligence or competence.

Migration Patterns

During the years in which slavery flourished in the South, fifteen million Africans were brought to this country from many parts of Africa. They brought with them rich traditions, languages, and cultures, which represented many different geographic regions of Africa as well as different nations and tribes.

The major migration of African Americans from the southern United States to northern states occurred between 1940 and 1970. During this migration African Americans generally settled in cities, where there was a great demand for unskilled labor.

Due to racial discrimination and segregation, many African Americans in cities have had unequal access to opportunities to achieve economic security. Therefore, many families have been unable to move out of areas of cities that tend to be known for higher rates of violence, bad housing, and poor health.

The Legacy of Slavery

The culture of African Americans has been defined through the experience of slavery and its aftermath. Africans came to this country with histories rich in culture and language and strong ties to family and community. These strong cultural roots have sustained families during difficult times and produced many important contributions to American culture and society.

The dehumanizing experiences of slavery in which human beings were bought and sold, families were separated, language and religion were discouraged, were followed by years of poor economic opportunity, racism, and discrimination. The legacy of these experiences for African Americans is evidenced in many ways, some of which affect the African Americans' attitudes about health care.

Spiritual Traditions

The church is an important social and spiritual institution in African American culture. African American churches often incorporate music and faith traditions that stem from a strong African heritage, as well as from the years in which religion and faith sustained Africans during slavery.

African American churches include a range of Catholic and Protestant sects. Many African Americans have begun to practice the Islam religion, the faith of Muslims.

Family

The extended family is a central institution in African American culture and may include "uncles" and "aunts" who are not blood relatives but who fulfill family roles. Elders in the family and community are respected and are often given decision-making authority. The extended family is a strong institution. Child-rearing responsibilities and medical decision making may be shared by grandparents. In addition, grandmothers may be the family delegates who make decisions about whether to accept a plan of care or a new health care provider.

Diet and Nutrition

Food is an integral part of African American culture. It is associated with family gatherings and the socialization of children. Some traditional foods may contribute to the genetic link between obesity and chronic illnesses, such as high blood pressure and diabetes. Care should be taken in discussion of diet and nutrition to communicate reasons for recommending dietary changes.

Attitudes and General Beliefs About Illness and Death

The experiences of slavery and racism have influenced the ways in which African Americans may relate to health care institutions in the following ways.

There is a history of African Americans having poor or nonexistent access to health care. This has led, for some, to a lack of trust that help will be available to them. This may result in a reluctance to seek health care.

This same history leads some families to believe that they will have to fight for their children's right to health care and that they cannot trust, automatically, that their children will receive the best of care. This can lead to what may appear to be overvigilance or questioning of medical advice and needs to be met with understanding and clear communication.

African Americans may be suspicious of research protocols or new treatments. This may stem from unethical medical experimentation such as the Tuskegee experiment in which, for four decades, African American men with syphilis were followed in a government-sponsored program but were denied any treatment. Clarifying informed consent is essential to engaging families in genuine partnerships with providers.

Implications for Providers

Cultural Courtesies   It is considered respectful, in meeting new patients, to use patient's full names and to call adults by Mr. or Mrs. The provider should attend to body language and tone of voice to ensure that respect is conveyed.

Communication Patterns and Value Orientation   The provider is encouraged to become acquainted with patients and their families and ask about their beliefs and experiences with the health care system.

The stress of vigilance regarding subtle or overt racism can create barriers to communication, as well as stress-related illness.

Traditional Medical Practices   Some families may rely on herbal medicines.

Other Issues Relevant to Hospitalization   African American attitudes and behavior toward providers and institutions may vary greatly depending on their socioeconomic status. However, some African Americans may feel that, regardless of their status, initial contact with and treatment by hospital staff is based initially on a negative stereotype. Therefore, it is very important that hospital staff treat every patient with the highest level of respect and courtesy.

Hair and skin care may require special combs or oils. Providers should ask what is needed.

References

Black, L. (1996). Families of African origin: An overview. In M. McGoldrick, J. Giordano, & J. K. Pearce (Eds.), *Ethnicity and family therapy.* New York: Guilford Press.

Fox, K. (1997, September 25). Inequities in health care closely correlated to race, income level. *Bay State Banner,* p. 9a.

Washington, H. (1997, October 26). Fear of medical care can become deadly. *EMERGE.*

Websites: *http://nativesearch.com/index.shtml* and *www.nativeweb.org* and *www.blackhealthnet.com*

Native American (North American Indian)

Introduction

This information is given as an introduction to a specific culture and is meant to help providers understand similarities and variations in cultural practices. Providers are cautioned not to overgeneralize or characterize all members of a cultural or ethnic group as alike. Factors to be considered in assessing a person's cultural identity and his or her actions or beliefs include individual characteristics, socioeconomic status, race, education, religion, age, gender; the stages, conditions, and adjustment to the migration experience; and whether the family came from a rural or urban area.

This information is about Native American traditions.

Country of Origin and Geographic Location

According to the 1990 United States census, there are two million Native Americans, comprising approximately five hundred different groups or "tribes." Native Americans live in both urban and rural areas throughout the United States. Many live in the 314 reservations located in all fifty states.

Native Americans are not a homogenous group; different tribes have their own distinct customs, cultures, and languages.

Some Native Americans prefer to be referred to as North American Indians, and others prefer to be called by their tribal names.

Language

There are many Native American languages, but the extent to which they are spoken varies widely. In many tribes the language has been forgotten, whereas in others everyone speaks it. It is through oral tradition that Native American cultures have been preserved. In recent years there has been a movement to preserve many Indian languages along with history, music, and art.

There are intergenerational differences in regard to the self-identification as "Indian." In addition, there are divergent beliefs about whether young people should have the opportunity to learn the tribal language.

Migration Patterns

In the 18th and 19th centuries, Indian tribes were forcibly relocated from traditional homelands to reservations, often thousands of miles away. Native Americans were settled into areas of the country not considered valuable by the American government at the time.

In the 1950s and 1960s, the U.S. government tried to move Native Americans from reservations to cities to promote opportunities for employment. This move resulted in social and health problems for the Native Americans, including an increase in alcoholism, associated with isolation from cultural support systems.

There are regional and tribal differences in patterns of migration. In some areas of the country, people leave the reservation for school or jobs and then return for periods of time. In other areas, there has been some recent migration back to traditional lands.

Cultural Repression

Three aspects of the history of the Native American experience are important to an understanding of current attitudes and cultural beliefs. First, in the late 19th Century millions of Indians died through warfare and forced migration to reservations. Second, many died as a result of diseases spread by Europeans, including smallpox and venereal disease. Last, when Native Americans were placed on reservations, the U.S. government required that all children attend boarding schools far from their families and community. In these schools, children were not permitted to use their own languages or learn about their native traditions. In effect, boarding schools led to whole generations of children losing their culture, their language, and their sense of identity.

The legacy of war, forced migration, and separation of children from their families is one of distrust and suspicion of authority still felt by many Native Americans.

Spiritual Traditions

Native Americans have "probably as many religious beliefs as there are tribes, each with sacred songs, dance, and prayers" (Kramer & Osborne, 1996). Indians may be members of traditional religions and/or any of the Christian traditions. In some parts of the country, the Native American Church is strong.

The practice of Native American religions was banned by the government in the 1800s. This legislation was only rescinded in 1979 through the Indian Freedom of Religion Act. Those practicing traditional Indian religion may be reluctant to discuss their religious beliefs or practices.

Family

American Indian cultures vary greatly in terms of how kinship is defined and structured. Each tribe decides who are members, with the rules varying among tribes. In some tribes the extended family may be the unit for decision making, whereas in others it could be the clan or another structure. Elders are generally highly respected.

Diet and Nutrition

For some Native Americans, dietary practices were formed through the government's program to provide commodity foods to those living on reservations. The current diet is generally rich in fat. This can lead to health problems such as high cholesterol and high blood pressure. Alcoholism is a major health problem in many Native American communities.

Attitudes and General Beliefs About Illness and Death

Traditional beliefs and practices generally focus on holistic approaches to health and well-being. Traditional medicine men may be consulted in times of illness for help with decision making and for domestic issues. Medicine men conduct healing ceremonies, which seek to help individuals regain harmony with their social and physical environment.

In general, traditional Native American beliefs about health and illness posit a strong relationship between physical and spiritual health. Healing ceremonies and dances may help patients regain spiritual balance, which is synonymous with improved health.

Implications for Providers

Cultural Courtesies   Providers should ask patients how they would like to be identified, for example, "American Indian," "Native American," or by a tribal name. Some Native Americans may be highly identified with a tribal tradition and others may not.

Communication Patterns and Value Orientation   There are generational differences in respect to attitudes about health and illness, as well as degrees of trust in hospitals and care providers.

- Although American Indians generally wear western clothing, this does not mean that they do not strongly identify with a Native American culture.

- Providers should ask about family structure, for example, who is expected to take part in decision making about medical care and home care procedures.

Traditional Medical Practices   Consultation with medicine men and participation in healing ceremonies may be important to Native American patients and their families.

- Medicine men are likely to treat spiritual distress or imbalance.

- Patients may wish to use herbal teas and other natural medicines to cure illness.

Other Issues Relevant to Hospitalization   Health care on reservations historically was provided through the Federal Indian Health Service, which ran hospitals and clinics that were free for Native Americans. Currently the government is turning control of the health services over to individual tribal communities.

References

Etta, C., Sulton, T., & Broken Nose, M. A. (1996). American Indian families: An overview. In M. McGoldrick, J. Giordano, & J. K. Pearce (Eds), *Ethnicity and family therapy.* New York: Guilford Press.

Hultkrantz, A. (1989). Health, religion and medicine in the world's religious traditions. In L. Sullivan (Ed.), *Healing and restoring in the world's religious traditions.* New York: Macmillan.

Kramer, J., & Osborne, B. (1996). American Indians. In J. G. Lipson, S. L. Dibble, & P. A. Minarik (Eds.), *Culture and nursing care: A pocket guide.* San Francisco: University of California San Francisco Nursing Press.

Weaver, H. (1998, May). Indigenous people in a multicultural society: Unique issues for human services. *Social Work, 431*(3), 203–211.

Puerto Rico

Introduction

This information is given as an introduction to a specific culture and is meant to help providers understand similarities and variations in cultural practices. Providers are cautioned not to overgeneralize or characterize all members of a cultural or ethnic group as alike. Factors to be considered in assessing a person's cultural identity and his or her actions or beliefs include individual characteristics, socioeconomic status, race, education, religion, age, gender; the stages, conditions, and adjustment to the migration experience; and whether the family came from a rural or urban area.

The following information is about Puerto Rican traditions and practices.

Country of Origin and Geographic Location

Puerto Rico is a commonwealth of the United States, located in the Caribbean Sea.

Language

Both Spanish and English are taught in schools in Puerto Rico. Most Puerto Ricans living in the continental United States speak both Spanish and English.

Migration Patterns

Puerto Ricans are U.S. citizens. Many families travel back and forth from the mainland to Puerto Rico. This has resulted in reinforcement of the Puerto Rican culture as well as the development of a bicultural identity.

Spiritual Traditions

Although the majority (75 percent) of Puerto Ricans are Roman Catholic, many are converting to Baptist, Pentecostal, Seventh Day Adventist, or the Jehovah's Witness churches. Other spiritual traditions include Espiritism and Santería.

Family

Familial relationships tend to be important in Puerto Rican culture. The family tends to be close-knit and emotionally and financially supportive. Often families that come from the island for medical treatment may not have this family support. Providers may be looked to as part of the extended support system.

Diet and Nutrition

The Puerto Rican diet consists of foods with their origins in Indian, Spanish, and African cultures. Rice and beans are the basic staples of the Puerto Rican diet. Many varieties of beans (for example, garbanzos, "frijoles negros," and "gandules") are used. Other common foods include tropical fruits, root vegetables (potatoes, "yautia," plantain, and ñame), fish, and meats. "Malta" is a malt-based soda that many people like. Sanjur (1995) writes that dietary trends practiced by Puerto Rican mothers include giving or withholding certain foods during illness, giving cleansing teas and coffee, and encouraging weight gain.

Attitudes and General Beliefs About Illness and Death

Puerto Ricans tend to live in close-knit communities; therefore, many cultural values and health traditions remain strong. Extended families are sources of support for the ill. Customs and rituals surrounding death are often aligned with the Roman Catholic, Espiritism, and Santería traditions.

Implications for Providers

Cultural Courtesies   Many people of Latin American descent prefer to be referred to as "Latino" rather than "Hispanic," yet it is more accurate to describe families by the area from which they come, for example, "Puerto Rican."

- Providers are generally seen as respected figures in Puerto Rican culture; however, traditional beliefs may conflict with the instructions of the provider.

- The patient or family may agree with the provider out of respect. This may not necessarily indicate that they intend to comply.

- Families will usually assist with most of the patient care. Because the extended family is the basis of their community, providers should discuss the care of the patient with the adult family members.

- The father or the oldest male is often considered to be the head of the family. Medical care should be discussed with him, if he is present; however, it is most often that the mother or grandmother will carry out the medical instructions.

Communication Patterns and Value Orientation   Lowering the eyes or avoiding direct eye contact is a sign of respect rather than distrust or fear.

- It is customary to shake hands when greeting.

- Puerto Ricans may stand in close groups when they are talking, and they may gesture with their hands.

- During a conversation, members of a group may interrupt one another. This would not be considered to be rude.

- In Latino culture, taking time to nurture personal relationships is considered more important than being on time. One may risk being late for an appointment to stop and talk with a friend. As with all families, the provider may want to explain the importance of being on time for appointments.

Traditional Medical Practices   Many traditional practices come from the Caribbean's African influence.

- A "curandero" or "espiritista" is a person who is believed to have spiritual powers for curing diseases and controlling spirits.

- A "botánica" is a resource store in the Latino community, where families can buy herbs and other more traditional remedies.

- Some Puerto Rican families may refer to the curandero, espiritista, or botánica before consulting a physician.

Other Issues Relevant to Hospitalization   Asthma may also be known as "fatiga." When a patient or parent says that the patient does not have asthma, they are often referring to the present tense, as in "I do not have asthma symptoms right now."

References

David Kennedy Center for International Studies. (1996). *Culturgrams: Puerto Rico.* Provo, UT: Brigham Young University.

Lynch, E. W., & Hanson, M. J. (Eds.). (1992). *Developing cross-cultural competencies.* Baltimore, MD: Paul H. Brookes Publishing Co.

Sanjur, D. (1995) *Hispanic foodways, nutrition and health.* Needham, MA: Allen & Bacon.

Chapter 8

Nationality-Independent Cultural Groups

Deaf or Hard-of-Hearing

Introduction

This information is given as an introduction to a specific culture and is meant to help providers understand similarities and variations in cultural practices. Providers are cautioned not to overgeneralize or characterize all members of a cultural or ethnic group as alike. Factors to be considered in assessing a person's cultural identity and his or her actions or beliefs include individual characteristics, socioeconomic status, race, education, religion, age, gender; the stages, conditions, and adjustment to the migration experience; and whether the family came from a rural or urban area.

The following information is about the traditions and practices of deaf or hard-of-hearing Americans.

Country of Origin and Geographic Location

The Deaf Community   There is great diversity among members of the deaf community. Deaf persons may affiliate as members of different communities, including those of persons from countries other than the United States, those of varying ethnic traditions, and those of specific religious traditions. The following information pertains to deaf American culture.

Approximately 10 percent of Americans have varying degrees of hearing loss, but not all are members of the deaf community. Members of the deaf community (of whom there are about one million in the United States) are united by the use of American Sign Language (ASL). Members of the deaf community do not view deafness as a "handicap" or as "pathological," but as a linguistic and cultural identity.

Hard-of-Hearing   Hard-of-hearing people have partial or no residual hearing. They may or may not know ASL. They choose to communicate through speech, speech reading, or assistive technology (hearing aids or other electronic devices). They may or may not be able to understand speech in one-on-one situations. Their own speech may or may not be difficult to understand.

Late-Deafened   The term "late-deafened" refers to people who became deaf after developing language. They may lose their hearing at any age, suddenly or over time. Some late-deafened people use sign language and may request an interpreter. They may also depend on more visual technology such as writing or electronic devices.

Language

There are many subpopulations of the U.S. deaf community. As spoken language varies from region to region, so does ASL.

The vast majority of deaf Americans share ASL as their primary language. American Sign Language is the fourth most frequently used language in the United States. It is a true language, not based on English.

If a deaf patient is visiting or recently emigrated from another country, it is unlikely that he or she will use ASL. Deaf people from Britain will likely use British Sign Language (BSL), just as a deaf person from Vietnam will speak VSL. Each language is unique.

Spiritual Traditions

Like the hearing population, deaf Americans may belong to any of the world's religions. In the United States, there are ministries and congregations for the deaf that offer services in ASL. Deaf patients and family members may appreciate consultation with deaf clergy.

Family

Approximately 90 percent of deaf children are born to hearing parents. Only 10 percent are born to deaf parents. Family dynamics between these two groups can often differ. Deaf parents who have deaf babies may be excited and pleased that their child will share their deaf identity. Hearing parents may often express grief or anger if their child is "hearing-impaired"; they may want to fix the condition in some way. Many hearing family members do not learn to sign, therefore severely limiting communication and bonding. Many deaf adults consider their community their family; they serve as support systems in time of illness and assist with decision making concerning health care issues.

Attitudes and General Beliefs About Illness and Death

Years of inadequate access to communication regarding health care may create a sense of wariness of health care professionals and the health care system. Deaf people's skills and abilities are often underestimated. Often deaf persons are not given the ability to participate in their own health care. As a result, they may lack knowledge of personal health history, illness, symptomatology, and medical terminology.

Implications for Providers

Cultural Courtesies   Providers should be aware of the deaf person's visual world. Attend to body language and facial expressions. Allow extra time for the assessment and interview. Working in two languages takes time.

Communication Patterns and Value Orientation   A common mistake is to assume that deaf persons are fluent in the language of the provider.

- Providers should ask the patient his or her primary language and how he or she wishes to communicate (that is, through a sign language interpreter or by writing notes).

- Providers should be aware that only 30 percent of speech is visible on the mouth; lip reading is not an accurate mode of communication.

- As with speakers of any foreign language, family members should not be used as interpreters.

- Providers should use eye contact and talk directly to the deaf person, not to the interpreter.

- The provider should keep his or her face clear of obstructions. Remove masks or scarves and keep hair out of the face when talking with a deaf or hard-of-hearing person.

- Greetings and leave taking are often accompanied by hugging.

- In order to get a deaf person's attention, one may tap him or her gently on the knee, shoulder, or forearm.

- Because storytelling is a large part of the deaf culture, a provider may elicit a lengthy, detailed, and very descriptive response to a question.

- Visual materials can help reinforce communication.

Other Issues Relevant to Hospitalization   Providers should not restrict a deaf person's hands or arms, remove a deaf person's eye wear, or cover his or her eyes.

- A teletypewriter machine (TTY) and a television with captioning may be helpful.

- Visual fire alarms should be provided when possible.

References

Ebert, D., & Heckerling, P. (1995). Communication with deaf patients: Knowledge, beliefs and practices of physicians. *Journal of the American Medical Association, 207*(3), 227–229.

Gannon, J. (1981). *Deaf heritage.* Silver Spring, MD: National Association for the Deaf.

Lane, H. (1992). *The mask of benevolence: Disabling the deaf community.* New York: Alfred Knopf.

Lane, H., Hoffmeister, R., & Bahan, B. (1996). *A journey into the deaf world.* San Diego, CA: Dawn Sign Press.

McEwan, E., & Anton-Culver, H. (1988). The medical communication of deaf patients. *Journal of Family Practice, 26*(3), 289–291.

Newport, E., & Meier, R. (1985). The acquisition of American Sign Language. In E. Slobin (Ed.), *The cross-linguistic study of language acquisition, Vol. 1: The Data.* Hillsdale, NJ: Erlbaum.

Padde, C., & Humphries, T. (1988). *Deaf in America: Voices from a culture.* Cambridge, MA: Harvard University Press.

Zazove, P., & Doukas, D. (1994). The silent healthcare crisis: Ethical reflections of healthcare for deaf and hard of hearing persons. *Family Medicine, 26,* 387–397.

Families with Gay or Lesbian Parents

Introduction

This information is given as an introduction to a specific culture and is meant to help providers understand similarities and variations in cultural practices. Providers are cautioned not to overgeneralize or characterize all members of a cultural or ethnic group as alike. Factors to be considered in assessing a person's cultural identity and his or her actions or beliefs include individual characteristics, socioeconomic status, race, education, religion, age, gender; the stages, conditions, and adjustment to the migration experience; and whether the family came from a rural or urban area.

The following information is about families with one or two gay or lesbian parents.

Demographics

An estimated six to fourteen million American children have at least one parent who is gay or lesbian (Gold et al., 1994; Perrin, 1996). It is difficult to obtain accurate statistics, as many homosexuals maintain their privacy.

Most gay or lesbian parents conceive their children in the context of a heterosexual relationship, before their homosexuality becomes evident. Some parents choose to remain in the marriage, and others separate or divorce. Many maintain their role as parent in a variety of custody, visitation, and family arrangements. Although many become single parents, others may co-parent in the context of a subsequent homosexual relationship.

In the last ten years, a growing number of gay and lesbian persons have chosen to become parents in the context of "singlehood" or a stable homosexual relationship. Gay men and lesbians have children through adoption, foster parenting, surrogacy arrangements, or alternative insemination via known or unknown donors (Gold et al., 1994).

Spiritual Traditions

Although some religious communities are welcoming of openly gay and lesbian persons (for example, Unitarian Universalist, United Church of Christ, Society of Friends), many religious groups condemn the homosexual lifestyle (for example, Orthodox Judaism, Islam, and Mormon). Other religious traditions are engaged in active dispute about allowing homosexuals to fully participate in church activities and leadership (for example, Episcopal, Lutheran, Presbyterian, and Roman Catholic).

Thus, gay and lesbian persons may be alienated from their religious traditions. If requested, the chaplain can refer families to gay-supportive local parishes and clergy and faith-specific gay and lesbian organizations.

A hospital chaplain can also provide nonjudgmental spiritual support or rituals such as baptism, the sacrament of the sick, and prayers at the time of death.

Research on Children of Gay or Lesbian Parents

Patterson's (1992) review of the research suggests that psychological health and social relationships of children of gay or lesbian parents are comparable to those of heterosexual families. The studies, although limited, show no significant differences in the development of moral maturity, gender identity, gender role, sexual orientation, and intelligence when compared with heterosexual families. The groups had comparable rates of psychiatric, behavioral, and emotional problems, but there was lower risk for parental sexual or physical abuse among children with gay or lesbian parents.

Discrimination

Although the civil liberties of most minorities in America have been protected by law, homosexuals are still vulnerable to violence and discrimination in most areas of life. Individuals who disclose a gay or lesbian identity risk rejection by family, peers, many organized religions, and the armed services. In the workplace and housing market, discrimination is not uncommon. In fact, hate crimes and violence against homosexuals are reported in many cities.

Ethnic groups have various attitudes about homosexuality. In some parts of the world, homosexuality is considered a crime punishable by imprisonment or death. In some cultures, family members who are identified as homosexual have been disowned or shunned. Gay and lesbian parents and their children may have difficulty maintaining ties with the ethnic group of their origin. In such cases, gay and lesbian families may create their own community or subculture in which gay or lesbian parents are common. On the other hand, some families may not disclose the structure of their family to those outside the household in order to maintain relationships with their cultural group.

Implications for Providers

Facilitating Disclosure   Perrin and Kulkin's (1996) survey of gay and lesbian parents revealed that many respondents worried about negative bias from health care providers or clinicians toward themselves or their children. This study showed that only 77 percent shared information about their family structure with their pediatrician.

The researchers suggest that disclosure about the family constellation is more likely when clinicians do not make assumptions about the identity or genders of the parents. Perrin (1996) and Gold et al. (1994) suggest that clinicians ask the following questions:

"Who else is taking care of this child with you?" or "Who else is in your household?" (Perrin & Kulkin, 1996, p. 362) or "To understand your child better, is there anything about your family that you think would be helpful for me to know?" (Gold et al., 1994, p. 356)

Office, clinic, and emergency forms are best written in gender-neutral language when referring to parents. Similarly, bulletin boards, magazines, and children's books in the waiting areas should picture nontraditional as well as traditional families with children (Perrin & Kulkin, 1996).

Family Structure   Because nontraditional families have a variety of constellations, providers should inquire about the family structure. Examples of helpful questions are, "Who are the primary decision makers in your family" or "Who would you like to include in conversations about hospital care, discharge teaching, and home care?" If the family requests that both partners be included, providers should honor that request in planning informational meetings or making treatment decisions. They can also assist both parents in obtaining hospital identification tags, if needed.

Other signs of respect include asking parents how they would like to be addressed by staff, such as co-parent or step-mother, as well as how they are referred to by their children (for example, "Daddy" and "Papa"). Adopt the language used or preferred. However, providers must not assume that this language applies to other nontraditional families.

Language or behaviors that diminish either parent, such as "Which of you is the real father?" should be avoided.

In addition, it is necessary to clarify what information can be passed along to other physicians, specialists, and care providers for the child, and, when appropriate, to document information about family structure in the medical record.

Other Issues Relevant to Hospitalization   In some families, only one parent may be able to provide consent for health care procedures.

- A number of states have legalized the co-adoption of children by same-sex parents. In such cases, both parents are authorized to provide consent. Providers should ask: "How do you handle legal consent forms for your child?" In nontraditional families, it is especially important to document information about guardianship and consent and to pass the information along to other providers as needed.

- Legal support for nontraditional families has increased in recent years; however, the precedents and laws governing custody differ from state to state. In some states, parents cannot adopt children if either is a homosexual. Custody and visitation issues can be reopened by a former spouse or extended family member if the parent's homosexuality was unknown at the time of the custody decision or if the family moves to another state (Gold et al., 1994). The provider should be sensitive to the concerns of parents regarding confidentiality and assess availability of support from extended family members.

- Nontraditional families have diverse histories and backgrounds. How a child was conceived or adopted is a private matter, that the family may not wish to discuss with multiple caregivers or with the child.

- Children also vary in the candor with which they share information about their family structure with peers, especially during adolescence. Providers should allow patients to disclose information as they wish, especially when peers are present.

Developmental Issues of Children   Extra social pressures affect children in gay or lesbian-headed families. For example, a young child's transition into school is often a time when families and children need support in explaining their family structure and events surrounding the child's birth to a wider community (Perrin & Kulkin, 1996).

Another difficult time is adolescence, when all children become more interested in their own developing sexuality and desire conformity with their peer group. It is common for children to be asked or teased about homosexuality by peers, based on their parent's lifestyle (Gold et al., 1994). Children are often reluctant to disclose their family arrangements in school. In these situations, health care providers, especially the pediatrician or nurse practitioner, may wish to offer these families an opportunity to discuss such special concerns or refer them to an appropriate support group for teens with gay or lesbian parents (Perrin & Kulkin, 1996).

References

D'Augelli, A. R., & Patterson, C. J. (Eds.). (1992). *Lesbian, gay, and bisexual identities over the lifespan.* New York: Oxford University Press.

Gold, M. A., Perrin, E. C., Futterman, O. F., & Friedman, S. B. (1994). Children of gay or lesbian families. *Pediatrics in Review, 15,*(9), 354–358.

Gottman, J. S. (1989). Children of gay and lesbian parents. *Marriage Family Review, 14,* 177–196.

Patterson, C. J. (1992). Children of lesbian and gay parents. *Child Development, 63,* 1025–1042.

Perrin, E. C., & Kulkin, H. (1996). Pediatric care for children whose parents are gay or lesbian. *Pediatrics, 97,* 629–635.

Case Study

Caribbean Culture

FROM THIS CASE STUDY ABOUT A FAMILY from a Caribbean culture, the staff learned about differences in gender roles and expectations; an "outsider's" skepticism of the U.S. health care system; the use of present-time versus future orientation; and the importance of involving extended family members. Our North American providers were not accustomed to these differences and benefitted from communication with a Haitian intermediary.

"Marie" was a nine-month-old baby girl born to Haitian parents. She was admitted to Children's Hospital shortly after she was born. Her medical diagnosis was very complicated: she required surgery, the placement of a gastrostomy tube, and several months' stay in the hospital. Marie's condition was not detected in utero, and the family was unprepared, distressed, and overwhelmed by Marie's condition and need for extensive care.

When Marie was admitted in the hospital, her parents and older brother lived with extended family nearby. Yet, shortly after Marie was hospitalized her mother and brother returned to Haiti. Marie's father stayed in the area and was, by default, considered Marie's primary caretaker. Marie's father, Mr. P, shared little personal information with the staff. Marie's nurses, applying the hospital's philosophy of "family centered care" and parental participation, became frustrated that Mr. P refused to take a more active role in his daughter's care. They became impatient with him, and he with them. The nurses expected Mr. P to bond with Marie, to become more attuned to the changes in her condition, and to learn the daily care he would have to provide at home. Of particular concern was his refusal to participate in Marie's plan of care. Mr. P further alienated the staff by making patronizing remarks toward the nursing staff and social workers, who were all women. Developing an alliance with Mr. P and planning care for Marie became increasingly difficult. He seemed to distrust the staff and the hospital system. When the nurses requested an interpreter to review the complex aspects of Marie's care, Mr. P haughtily refused the offer.

Marie's health care team—nurses, doctors, social workers, and psychiatrists—developed a working plan to understand the cultural nuances of Mr. P's behavior. The social worker made a referral to a social service agency with which Mr. P was familiar and comfortable. Informational literature about Haitian culture was put in the patient's chart. A cultural consultant came to talk with the team about cultural traditions that might have an impact on Mr. P's behavior. Through this discussion it became evident that the issues central to this particular situation were

- Differences in gender roles and expectations (men in Haiti not being comfortable taking orders from women and their discomfort with child care)

- Distrust of the U.S. health care provider and medical system (sense of entitlement to services)

- Present-time orientation (tendency to focus on today's issues and not plan for the future)

- Importance of the extended family (which took the mother to Haiti and left the father to ask aunts to help with Marie's care)

In Haitian culture, women are the child-care providers. The husbands are the financial providers. In this situation, a role reversal existed; Mr. P suddenly found himself in the role more typical of his wife, having to be Marie's care provider. Also, he was not able to work, losing his masculine role of financial provider.

Because the nursing staff were all women, he was uncomfortable taking direction from them. On a daily basis the nurses asked him to be more involved with Marie's care, duties usually delegated to mothers, aunts, and grandmothers. Mr. P's reaction was to ignore their requests. When planning for Marie's discharge, his role as financial provider and primary decision maker was eliminated: he was not able to bring Marie home to his own apartment but rather to that of an aunt. This lack of ability to provide arose again when it was clear that Marie would need assistance from many community services.

Mr. P's knowledge of the U.S. health care system was extensive. He demanded services beyond what was necessary or even available to Marie. He seemed frustrated by the limitations of the system (such as unavailability of twenty-four-hour care) and at the same time resented having to provide financial information in order to qualify for services.

Mr. P's sense of time orientation was different from that of the nurses. He seemed relaxed and not able to see the need to perform procedures in a timely manner, such as giving medications or feedings. Haitians have a present-time orientation and may not view future-oriented tasks or time schedules as important as the present.

Mr. P seemed to resent the assumption that he was the sole care provider, while the aunts and grandmother were not included in the plan of care. Yet he felt unable to ask them himself, due to his need to be the primary decision maker and authority figure. In essence, he needed help and was either afraid to ask for it or resented needing assistance with Marie.

Armed with knowledge of the cultural background of the patient and family, the health care team was able to see Mr. P's behavior as less personal and offensive. The health care team sent a direct invitation to Marie's aunts and grandmother to be involved in her care. Mr. P was then able to tell them what he knew about Marie's care, putting him in the role of authority figure while ensuring assistance for Marie. The nurses drew up a calendar to help Mr. P and the family work on goals for discharge. Mr. P became engaging, goal oriented, and—while somewhat disappointed in the lack of extensive services for Marie—accepting of the service plan.

Part Two

Religious Traditions

Chapter 9

Religion and Spirituality

The Department of Pastoral Care and the Family Education Program at Children's Hospital, Boston, have developed the information sheets in Chapter 10 to assist health care providers working with families from various religious backgrounds. These sheets provide an introduction to specific religious traditions and are meant to help providers understand similarities and variations in religious practice.

Providers are cautioned not to overgeneralize or characterize all members of a religious group as alike. Factors to be considered in assessing a person's spiritual identity, practice, and beliefs include: age, sex, ethnic group, faith community, family structure, life experience, and individual characteristics.

Special Issues for Providers

Demographics

The 1990 Gallup poll showed that 96 percent of Americans believe in God, and 58 percent say that religion is very important in their lives. A number participate in organized religious traditions. A much smaller proportion of physicians (64 percent) and mental health professionals (33 percent) say that they believe in God (Bergin & Payne, 1990; Maugans & Wadland, 1991). Reliable statistical data on spirituality is more difficult to obtain, given the lack of consensus regarding its definition (Dyson et al., 1997).

Spirituality Versus Religion

Most people, including young children, are spiritual. Some people are religious. Spirituality and religion are neither identical nor synonymous.

Religion is typically experienced within a social institution with commonly shared traditions, sacred texts, beliefs, and worship practices. Religious institutions usually have a governing structure with designated leaders.

Spirituality, on the other hand, is that part of each person that searches for purpose, meaning, worth, and wonder, often in quest of an ultimate value or the holy. A person's spirituality may be an individual or social matter and may find expression in a wide variety of practices (for example, vocation, wilderness experiences, contemplation, art, meditation, prayer, and religious worship). Spirituality enhances one's inner resources and serenity.

Language

People may use secular language (for example, "I just cannot understand why this is happening to me") or religious language (for example, "I cannot pray or go to synagogue since my child got sick") when talking about spiritual concerns. Providers should match terminology with that of the patient.

Benefits

Medical research suggests that a patient's spirituality and religion can have beneficial effects on his or her general health, including lowered blood pressure, improved quality of life, and increased survival rates (Matthews & Larson, 1993, 1995, 1998). For some patients, religion or spirituality may be key coping mechanisms during illness or hospitalization. It may be a primary way to find meaning from the illness or to find hope, forgiveness, or guilt in the situation (Dyson et al., 1977). For those in a faith community, religion can facilitate relationships that function as extended family and social supports.

Patients often wish to discuss their spiritual or religious needs. One study found that 77 percent of patients wanted their physicians to consider their spiritual needs, while 68 percent reported that their physicians had never discussed the topic (King & Bushwick, 1994).

Facilitating Discussion About Spiritual Matters

A person's ultimate beliefs and relationship with the holy are often considered very private matters. In North America, most people are not accustomed to discussing such things openly with strangers. Discussion of such sensitive matters is facilitated when the provider has established a relationship of trust with the patient and has conveyed respect for spiritual concerns. The discussion of spiritual concerns usually enhances the patient-provider relationship.

The provider is encouraged to inquire about the family's spiritual needs near the end of an initial interview. Perhaps the topic can be introduced by saying: "We know that illness can be very stressful. Many families find their faith or spiritual beliefs a source of strength or comfort during a hospital stay. I'm wondering if your spirituality or religion is important to you?" If the patient or family says "yes," these questions follow naturally:[*]

"Do you follow a particular religious tradition or spiritual path?" If the answer is yes, "Would you like a visit from your own clergy or a hospital chaplain during your stay?" If the answer is yes, "Would you like to include that person in the conversation when it comes time to make an important treatment decision?"

Some other possible questions include the following:

- "Are there religious customs or spiritual practices that are important to you, but likely to be disrupted during this hospital stay or illness?"

- "Are there ways that we can help you maintain your spiritual strength or routine during this stay (for example, worship opportunities, medals, devotional materials, kosher meals, Sabbath candles, communion, baptism, prayer rug, and so forth)?"

- "How does your faith influence the way you think about this illness?"

If the patient or family says that religion or spirituality is *not* important, the following questions may be asked:

- "Do you find strength and support in other areas of your life?"

- "Are there ways we can facilitate this during your stay in the hospital?"

---

[*] These questions were adapted from L. Carpenito, *Nursing Diagnosis: Application to Clinical Practice* (7th ed.). New York: Lippincott Williams & Wilkins, 1997.

Offering Spiritual Support

The provider does not need to be a person of faith (or of the same faith as the patient) to attend to the person's spiritual needs. Providers should consult with a chaplain who will support the patient and family in their chosen tradition and help interpret it to the rest of the care team. Providers and hospital chaplains may facilitate spiritual or religious observance in the hospital setting, if desired.

If the patient expresses an interest in a religious practice, the provider should ask how well the practice is meeting his or her needs. If it is not, the services of a chaplain should be offered.

When to Call a Chaplain

Call the chaplain if

- The patient or family requests to see a chaplain or member of the clergy;

- The patient or family wishes sacramental, devotional, or other religious rituals;

- The patient is dying;

- The patient or family wishes to consider a medical decision from a faith perspective;

- Symptoms of spiritual distress are noted;

- The patient or family identify spirituality or religion as a significant source of strength or comfort;

- The patient or family raises religious objections to the proposed plan for care or autopsy;

- Religious or spiritual beliefs of the patient or family appear pathological or problematic;

- A provider requests more information about a religious tradition and its relevance to the hospital setting;

- Special accommodations are needed for religious or cultural practices during care, education, or discharge; or

- An in-depth spiritual assessment would be helpful to providers.

References

Bergin, A., & Payne, I. (1990). Religiosity of psychotherapists: A national survey. *Journal of Psychotherapy, 27,* 3–7.

Dein, S. (1997). Does being religious help or hinder coping with chronic illness? A critical literature review. *Palliative Medicine, 11,* 291–308.

Dyson, J., Cobb, M., & Forman, D. (1997). The meaning of spirituality: A literature review. *Journal of Advanced Nursing, 26,* 1183–1188.

King, D. E., & Bushwick, B. (1994). Beliefs and attitudes of hospital inpatients about faith healing and prayer. *Journal of Family Practice, 39,* 349–352.

Maugans, T., & Wadland, W. (1991). Religion and family medicine: A survey of physicians and patients. *Journal of Family Practice, 32*(2), 210–213.

Matthews, D. A., & Larson, D. B. (1993, 1995, 1998). *The faith factor: An annotated bibliography of clinical research on spiritual subjects* (Vols. 1–3). Washington, DC: National Institute of Health Care Research.

Chapter 10

Religions

Buddhism

Introduction

This information is given as an introduction to a specific religious tradition and is meant to help providers understand similarities and variations among religious practices. Providers are cautioned not to overgeneralize or characterize all members of a religious group as alike. In fact, a person's spiritual and religious profile is unique and can be determined only when trust has been established and open-ended assessment questions have been asked.

The provider is encouraged to inquire about the family's spiritual needs near the end of an initial interview. Perhaps the topic can be introduced by saying: "We know that illness can be very stressful. Many families find their faith or spiritual beliefs a source of strength or comfort during a hospital stay. I'm wondering if your spirituality or religion is important to you?" If the patient or family says "yes," these questions follow naturally:*

"Do you follow a particular religious tradition or spiritual path?" If the answer is yes, "Would you like a visit from your own clergy or a hospital chaplain during your stay?" If the answer is yes, "Would you like to include that person in the conversation when it comes time to make an important treatment decision?"

Some other possible questions include the following:

- "Are there religious customs or spiritual practices that are important to you, but likely to be disrupted during this hospital stay or illness?"

---

* These questions were adapted from L. Carpenito, *Nursing Diagnosis: Application to Clinical Practice* (7th ed.). New York: Lippincott Williams & Wilkins, 1997.

107

- "Are there ways that we can help you maintain your spiritual strength or routine during this stay (for example, worship opportunities, medals, devotional materials, kosher meals, Sabbath candles, communion, baptism, prayer rug, and so forth)?"

- "How does your faith influence the way you think about this illness?"

When making an assessment, additional factors to consider include age, gender, ethnic group, developmental stage, family structure, faith community, life experiences, psychosocial history, and individual characteristics. Providers should consult the hospital chaplain for assistance with an assessment.

The following information sheet is about Buddhist practices and traditions.

In Brief

- Buddhism originated in Nepal in the 6th Century B.C. and spread through much of Asia.

- There are many different kinds of Buddhism. Each has its own style and practice. The two major divisions are Mahayana (including Tibetan, Zen, and Pure Land) and Theravada.

- Buddhism is practiced in many different cultures and has many local variations. Some people practice Buddhism in conjunction with Christianity or Judaism.

- Buddhists accept responsibility for the ways they exercise their freedoms in life. The underlying principles, as taught by Buddhism's founder Siddhartha, are the four noble truths: (1) suffering is an important part of life; (2) suffering is caused by selfish craving; (3) this suffering can be brought to an end, (4) which will bring true happiness (Magida, 1996).

- Resolution lies in the practice of the eight-fold path. The eight-fold path refers to the right view or understanding, right thought, right speech, right action, right livelihood, right effort, right mindfulness, and right meditation.

- Buddhists believe that happiness comes from changing oneself from the inside to develop generosity, integrity, and self-knowledge. For many this is the way to enlightenment and also rebirth.

Place of Worship

Buddhists worship in a temple.

Clergy

Monks, nuns, and, in some places, ministers or priests serve the needs of the people.

Holy Days

Buddhists may observe the following holy days: January 1, January 16, February 15, March 21, April 8, May 21, June 15, August 1, August 23, December 8, and December 31.

Religious Observance in the Hospital Setting

Worship   Worship includes silent meditation, chanting, an offering of incense, and a talk by clergy. Buddhists may use an "ouzo" (similar to a rosary) to facilitate the saying of prayers. In Buddhism, worship is the acknowledgment of an ideal. This ideal is not seen as personified, such as a particular God, but as a state of being. For some, being able to have an altar with a small Buddha statue, a candle, incense, some water, and fresh fruit or flowers might be important. In the hospital setting, an electric candle or electric incense burner can be substituted. Providers should take care not to disturb or handle such items in the course of care or housekeeping.

Dietary Needs   Many, but not all, Buddhists are strict vegetarians. Some holy days include fasting.

Care of the Sick   *Pastoral Care.* Buddhist patients and families typically do not expect to see Buddhist clergy during hospitalization. Clergy may be consulted at or around the time of death. The family can provide the name of local clergy of their particular Buddhist denomination, language, and culture.

Prayer. Prayer in Buddhism is not a petition to a specific god but rather a tool for cleansing one's consciousness. Patients may bring a picture of the Buddha to the hospital room to facilitate meditation. Family and friends may chant to help create peace of mind and to create an atmosphere of positive energy and tranquility in which the patient can relax. If chanting is disturbing to other patients in a shared room, the hospital chapel or a private consultation room may be offered.

Treatment. If life can be prolonged for the cultivation of understanding, compassion, and joy for others and oneself, any treatment is justified. If the patient is beyond recovery and mindfulness, the family may be prepared for death.

The use of medication is welcomed when it helps to heal the body or facilitates the comfort of the friends and family supporting the patient, who wish not to see the patient suffer. The desire for medication to ease pain and suffering is balanced with the desire for a clear mind. Because terminal illness is seen as a unique opportunity to reflect on life's most ultimate meanings, refusal of medication is common.

Special Concerns   *Death.*   Death is seen as a process in the cyclical continuum, which includes birth, sickness, old age, death, rebirth, sickness, old age, death, and so on. Because death is associated with rebirth, great importance is attributed to the state of the person's mind, which should be calm and clear. This means that serene surroundings are important to the patient and family. No formal rituals are customary at the time of death. The family may wish to contact a monk who will pray for the deceased. Prayers do not need to be performed in the presence of the body. Routine postmortem care is generally acceptable. In most Buddhist countries, cremation is performed.

Autopsy.   In general, Buddhism does not oppose autopsies, blood transfusions, or transplants. Many Tibetan Buddhists believe that the dead body should not be cut or embalmed until three days have passed.

References

Council of Churches of Greater Springfield and the Visiting Nurse Hospice of Pioneer Valley. (1995). *Knowing my neighbor: Religious beliefs and cultural traditions at times of illness and death.* Springfield, MA: Council of Churches.

Eschleman, M. J. (1992, November). Death with dignity. *Today's O.R. Nurse,* pp. 19–23.

Kirkwood, N. (1995). *Hospital handbook on multiculturalism and religion.* Harrisburg, PA: Moorehouse Publishing.

Magida, A. J. (Ed.). (1996). Buddhism. *How to be a perfect stranger.* Woodstock, NY: Jewish Lights Publishing.

Websites: *www.fas.harvard.edu/pluralsm,   www.buddhanet.net,*   and *www.dharmanet.org*

Church of Jesus Christ of Latter-Day Saints (Mormon)

Introduction

This information is given as an introduction to a specific religious tradition and is meant to help providers understand similarities and variations among religious practices. Providers are cautioned not to overgeneralize or characterize all members of a religious group as alike. In fact, a person's spiritual and religious profile is unique and can be determined only when trust has been established and open-ended assessment questions have been asked.

The provider is encouraged to inquire about the family's spiritual needs near the end of an initial interview. Perhaps the topic can be introduced by saying: "We know that illness can be very stressful. Many families find their faith or spiritual beliefs a source of strength or comfort during a hospital stay. I'm wondering if your spirituality or religion is important to you?" If the patient or family says "yes," these questions follow naturally:*

"Do you follow a particular religious tradition or spiritual path?" If the answer is yes, "Would you like a visit from your own clergy or a hospital chaplain during your stay?" If the answer is yes, "Would you like to include that person in the conversation when it comes time to make an important treatment decision?"

Some other possible questions include the following:

- "Are there religious customs or spiritual practices that are important to you, but likely to be disrupted during this hospital stay or illness?"

- "Are there ways that we can help you maintain your spiritual strength or routine during this stay (for example, worship opportunities, medals, devotional materials, kosher meals, Sabbath candles, communion, baptism, prayer rug, and so forth)?"

- "How does your faith influence the way you think about this illness?"

When making an assessment, additional factors to consider include age, gender, ethnic group, developmental stage, family structure, faith community, life experiences, psychosocial history, and individual characteristics.

---

* These questions were adapted from L. Carpenito, *Nursing Diagnosis: Application to Clinical Practice* (7th ed.). New York: Lippincott Williams & Wilkins, 1997.

Providers should consult the hospital chaplain for assistance with an assessment.

The following information is about Mormon practices and traditions.

In Brief

- Although many Mormon beliefs are distinctive, Mormons consider themselves Christian.

- The Church of Jesus Christ of Latter-day Saints was founded in 1830 by Joseph Smith, Jr., who was instructed by an angel to unearth a set of golden tablets with religious instruction, now known as the Book of Mormon.

- Following Smith's death, Brigham Young led the community west, fleeing persecution through the states of Ohio, Missouri, Illinois, Mississippi, Iowa, Nebraska, and Wyoming—finally settling in Utah and other western states.

- The western United States currently have the largest concentration of Mormons.

- The Book of Mormon is the source of the group's nickname. Although "Mormon" is not the correct name of the Church, it is not offensive. Most members refer to themselves as Latter-day Saints or LDS.

- In 1996, the church had 10 million members worldwide. It is one of the fastest growing religious traditions in Central and South America and has an expanding membership all over the world.

- Another much smaller group with Mormon roots calls itself the Reorganized Church of Jesus Christ of Latter Day Saints. They refer to themselves as "Saints" or "RLDS." The two churches distinguish themselves from one another and have different beliefs. The opinions of the Reorganized Church of Jesus Christ of Latter Day Saints are not given here. (See *www.rlds.org.*)

- The primary scriptures for Latter-day Saints are the King James Version of the Bible, the Book of Mormon, the Doctrine of Covenants, and the Pearl of Great Price.

Place of Worship

Churches are used for Sunday worship and weekly activities, and temples are used by the most observant for marriages and other sacred events.

Clergy

There are no professional clergy. Home teachers are the usual providers of pastoral care in the hospital setting. The bishop is the presiding local leader, with the assistance of men in the church who have been ordained to two levels of nonprofessional priesthood. Leadership of the national church is provided by a president (with two advisors) and a Council of Twelve Apostles from its headquarters in Salt Lake City, Utah.

Holy Days

Sunday is set aside for worship. Family Home Evening, usually on Mondays, is a time when the family shares in religious instructions, recreational activities, and prayer. Special holy days are Christmas (December 25) and Easter (in March or April).

Religious Observance in the Hospital Setting

Worship   Members typically have a Bible, Book of Mormon, or other scriptures at their bedside for daily reading and reflection. They may wish a nurse to obtain them from the chaplain's office if they have not brought their own from home.

Each member of the LDS church has a designated home teacher who visits on a regular basis. During times of illness or other problems, these members of the local congregation will make regular hospital visits, offer special prayers for the patient's welfare, perform the priesthood anointing of the sick, or the sacrament of the Lord's Supper (communion). The hospital chaplain facilitates the ministry of these lay visitors who function in clergy roles.

A member who is hospitalized away from home may wish the chaplain to contact the local Mormon congregation to provide a visitor for support and spiritual care. The "transient bishop" coordinates the care of persons from out of town.

Dietary Needs   Latter-day Saints abstain from tobacco, alcohol, coffee, tea, and illicit drugs. Some refrain from drinking caffeinated sodas.

Care of the Sick   *Treatment.* Mormons are very open to state-of-the-art medical treatment. The individual is the primary decision maker, in consultation with the family, the physician, qualified elder of the church, and other relevant professionals.

Special Concerns   *Clothing.* Faithful Mormons wear a religious undergarment not unlike long underwear, with short sleeves and legs to knee length. Exposing the garment is unacceptable, so Mormons are excused from wearing it when a hospital gown is needed for medical reasons. Because it is associated with faithfulness and divine protection from illness, clinical staff should be sensitive to those who desire the spiritual comfort of wearing it in the hospital setting. Such patients should be provided both hospital gowns and pants or the opportunity to bring pajamas from home to ensure modesty.

Birth. The ceremony for blessing and naming a newborn baby typically happens in church on the first Sunday of each month. Children are baptized by immersion in water at the age of eight. Infant baptisms are not done and never observed in the hospital setting. Persons with a developmental age of less than eight need not be baptized; their spiritual well-being is assured.

Social Services and Discharge Planning. The Church of Jesus Christ of Latter-day Saints has a monthly fast to raise money for the needy and has an organized system to provide assistance for those in need. Because local congregations have a strong belief in rendering service, they are generally very willing to provide cooked meals, transportation, assistance with chores, respite care, and financial assistance to families with illness and should be considered as a key resource for social services and discharge planning. This generosity applies to Mormon patients from out of town, who can often receive support from local congregations or the transient bishop.

Family Planning and Procreation. The Mormon community is known for its traditional views of the family. The bonds of marriage are considered sacred and eternal. Sexual intercourse among unmarried couples and homosexuality are subject to church discipline.

The Mormon community has consistently opposed elective abortion, except in situations in which the mother's life is in danger or the fetus is clearly nonviable or seriously defective.

Generally speaking, reproductive technologies that assist married couples and maintain the genetic link between child and both married parents are acceptable.

Care at the End of Life. The church supports families' thoughtful choices regarding care at the end of life. Because Mormons have a strong belief in life after death, they are willing to discuss Do Not Resuscitate (DNR) and redirection or withdrawal of care.

"No unreasonable means" are required by the church to prolong life when dying has become inevitable. "Unreasonable" is left to the discernment of the patient and family and medical team. Families may wish to take the decision to prayer and fasting and to consult with an elder of the church. Active euthanasia is prohibited.

Blessing of the Sick. There are no "last rites" in this tradition; however, patients may request the blessing of the sick during illness. Two elders of the church anoint the head of the sick person with consecrated olive oil and lay their hands on the patient's head while saying a special prayer for healing. The nurse may contact the chaplain's office to arrange for such a blessing. Privacy may be requested for this ritual.

Organ Transplantation. The church does not prohibit organ donation or transplantation.

Death. Mormons believe that at the time of death, a person's spirit separates from the body and returns to God, the giver of all life. The identity of a person is eternal and is reunited with others who have died before them. While grief is present, death is also seen as a transition to better things, rather than an ultimate loss. Family members may ask the dying patient to deliver fond messages to loved ones who have passed through death.

Autopsy. Autopsy is permitted. Some may desire that any organs removed during autopsy be replaced before burial.

Burial Customs. The decision to bury or cremate is left to the family. A funeral and burial service involves the faith community. Faithful Mormons are buried in their ritual temple attire.

References

Bush, L. E., Jr. (1993). *Health and medicine among the Latter-day Saints.* New York: Crossroads Publishing.

Harris-Albert, D. (Ed.). (1995). *The Latter-day Saints tradition: Religious beliefs and health care decisions.* Chicago: Park Ridge Center for the Study of Health, Faith and Ethics.

Magida, A. J. (Ed.). (1996). Latter-day Saints. *How to be a perfect stranger.* Woodstock, NY: Jewish Lights Publishing.

Website: *www.mormons.org*

First Church of Christ, Scientist (Christian Science)

Introduction

This information is given as an introduction to a specific religious tradition and is meant to help providers understand similarities and variations among religious practices. Providers are cautioned not to overgeneralize or characterize all members of a religious group as alike. In fact, a person's spiritual and religious profile is unique and can be determined only when trust has been established and open-ended assessment questions have been asked.

The provider is encouraged to inquire about the family's spiritual needs near the end of an initial interview. Perhaps the topic can be introduced by saying: "We know that illness can be very stressful. Many families find their faith or spiritual beliefs a source of strength or comfort during a hospital stay. I'm wondering if your spirituality or religion is important to you?" If the patient or family says "yes," these questions follow naturally:*

"Do you follow a particular religious tradition or spiritual path?" If the answer is yes, "Would you like a visit from your own clergy or a hospital chaplain during your stay?" If the answer is yes, "Would you like to include that person in the conversation when it comes time to make an important treatment decision?"

Some other possible questions include the following:

- "Are there religious customs or spiritual practices that are important to you, but likely to be disrupted during this hospital stay or illness?"

- "Are there ways that we can help you maintain your spiritual strength or routine during this stay (for example, worship opportunities, medals, devotional materials, kosher meals, Sabbath candles, communion, baptism, prayer rug, and so forth)?"

- "How does your faith influence the way you think about this illness?"

When making an assessment, additional factors to consider include age, gender, ethnic group, developmental stage, family structure, faith community, life experiences, psychosocial history, and individual characteristics.

---

* These questions were adapted from L. Carpenito, *Nursing Diagnosis: Application to Clinical Practice* (7th ed.). New York: Lippincott Williams & Wilkins, 1997.

Providers should consult the hospital chaplain for assistance with an assessment.

The following information is about Christian Science practices and traditions.

In Brief

- The First Church of Christ, Scientist, was founded in 1866 by Mary Baker Eddy, who was personally healed of an injury while reading a passage in the Bible about Jesus' powers of healing. She believed she had rediscovered the system of healing that Jesus used.

- Ms. Eddy established the Church of Christ, Scientist, now known as the "Mother Church" in Boston, Massachusetts, in 1879.

- Christian Science is based on a belief in "God as the all-loving Father-Mother, Christ Jesus as His Son, and individuals as God's children or spiritual reflection. Because God is understood to be all-good and the only reality of existence, evil (and illness) is regarded as fundamentally unreal and able to be overcome. Christian Scientists regard Christian Science as the spiritual laws of God by which Jesus healed" (Jones, 1998).

- Christian Scientists typically refuse most medical care in preference for that of a Christian Science practitioner.

- There are an estimated 2,200 Christian Science churches in seventy-four countries. The church is centered in Boston, Massachusetts.

- A complete explanation of Christian Science, including its healing practice, is found in *Science and Health with Key to the Scriptures*, by Mary Baker Eddy.

Place of Worship

Worship takes place in a Christian Science Church or in societies. The Christian Science Reading Rooms, often located in busy shopping areas, are centers for Christian Science prayer, for purchasing Mary Baker Eddy's writings, and for researching topics related to Christian Science.

Clergy

Christian Science does not have ordained clergy. Lay readers, selected by each local congregation, conduct church services. Christian Science practitioners are men and women who work full-time as healers in their communities. "They claim no personal healing power, but pray to recognize

God's ever-present love and all-power on behalf of the patient" (Jones, 1998).

Holy Days

Christian Scientists do not celebrate special holy days. Public worship services take place on Sundays. Testimony meetings are on Wednesday evenings.

Religious Observance in the Hospital Setting

Worship   Specific daily prayer is fundamental to the practice of Christian Science. Christian Scientists believe that this scientific approach to prayer yields practical results, such as freedom from stress, guidance in daily decisions, and physical healing. Privacy for daily prayers in the hospital setting is appreciated.

Many members read from the Bible and Eddy's *Science and Health* on a daily basis.

Communion is seen as "ongoing devotion to understanding God and living according to Jesus' teachings and works. It is specifically observed twice a year as silent prayer at church service" (Jones, 1998). Christian Scientists do not have a ceremony using bread and juice or wine.

Baptism is considered an ongoing process of spiritual renewal. There is no specific ritual in a hospital setting.

Dietary Needs   Christian Scientists typically abstain from alcohol, tobacco, medications, and illicit drugs. Many do not drink tea or coffee.

Care of the Sick   *Pastoral Care.* Christian Scientists generally pray independently. If further assistance is needed, a Christian Science practitioner may be called to provide additional prayer. "Practitioners treat all types of conditions, including physical ailments, injuries, anxiety, stress, as well as mental illness and addictive behaviors. Depending on the needs in each case, practitioners make bedside visits, consult over the phone, or see patients in their office" (Jones, 1998). The hospital chaplain can find a local Christian Science practitioner, when requested.

If a Christian Scientist elects Western medical treatment, the Christian Science practitioner normally withdraws and will no longer give specific treatment. This is to ensure that the patient is not subjected to opposing approaches.

Prayer. When Christian Scientists do get sick, they approach the healing of physical and emotional conditions exclusively through prayer. When the illness is treated in this way, Christian Scientists believe that spiritual healing (which includes physical healing) results.

Treatment. Christian Scientists respect the work of medical professionals; however, they typically rely on spiritual treatment rather than Western medical care. They will utilize obstetricians or certified midwives for childbirth. They might use orthopaedic surgeons to set broken bones, dentists for care of their teeth, and optometrists for eyeglasses.

Christian Scientists comply with mandatory physical exams and vaccinations, as well as quarantine laws for themselves and their children. Choice of care in each situation is an individual decision.

Christian Scientists rarely participate in medical research.

Special Concerns   Christian Scientists who choose traditional Western medicine may be unfamiliar with medical terminology, procedures, or the health care system. They may require reassurance and additional teaching.

Christian Scientists expect to participate in decision making about their care. They may wish to consult a Christian Science practitioner prior to undertaking any medical treatment.

Because Christian Scientists rely on spiritual treatment for health care, they may not be able to provide a documented medical history. However, they could give a general oral summary.

Christian Scientists who choose traditional Western medicine may experience disapproval from family members who prefer a spiritual approach. The provider is encouraged to inquire about the impact such a decision may have on the patient's family or social support systems.

Pain Management. Christian Scientists often refuse standard palliative care that includes pain medications, IV fluids, back rubs or massages, application of heat or ice, or use of a thermometer; however, "if an individual chooses to alleviate pain medically, this is not seen as precluding healing through prayer" (Jones, 1998). The choice to use pain medications may elicit spiritual distress on the part of the patient or family members, as this is not a customary practice among Christian Scientists.

Insurance Coverage. Christian Scientists make their own choices about insurance coverage. Many have hospital indemnity policies with a Christian Science rider. This would allow them to have Christian Science care and treatment; however, some Christian Scientists may not choose to have medical insurance, as they typically do not plan to use it (Jones, 1998).

Medical Treatment of Children. Christian Scientists commonly choose spiritual treatment for themselves and their children. However, should they choose to seek care in a hospital setting, they would generally accept the provider's medical diagnosis or treatment plan.

The courts have held that competent adult Christian Scientists can refuse medical care, even if it results in their own death; however, parents cannot refuse medically indicated treatment for a child when the child's life is in danger. A court order may be sought to enforce treatment for a child. Legal consultation should be sought with the hospital's Office of Legal Counsel in such situations.

If a court order is warranted, providers should inform the parents and offer them the opportunity to articulate their beliefs to the judge. They may wish to have spiritual and legal advocates present at the time. A member of the Christian Science community would be the preferable spiritual advocate, or the hospital chaplain can serve in that role.

Spiritual Distress. Choosing traditional medical care may elicit spiritual distress in a patient or family because it is so different from their religious practices. Even persons who are not currently active in Christian Science but who were raised in that tradition may have vestigial values, concerns, and expectations that have an impact on their health care. Contact with a member of the Christian Science community or the services of a Protestant chaplain may be offered.

Care at the End of Life. There are a number of privately maintained facilities where Christian Science nurses provide non-medical care. The providers offer spiritual encouragement and practical physical care. Such care does not include surgery, radiation, physical therapy, or medications. Analgesics would not be provided.

Do Not Resuscitate (DNR)/Redirection of Care. Because Christian Scientists generally rely on spiritual treatment instead of Western medical care, they generally forego all life-sustaining options. "They would not be inclined to passively accept the inevitability of death due to their reliance on God's healing power in all situations" (Jones, 1998).

Organ Donation. There are no restrictions against organ donation, although Christian Scientists have not typically donated organs.

Autopsy. Autopsies are permissible. Christian Scientists usually decline autopsy, except in instances when death is sudden. When possible, it is preferred that another female handle female bodies.

References

Eddy, M. B. (1994). *Science and health with key to the scriptures: Writings of Mary Baker Eddy.* Boston: Christian Science Publishing Society.

Jones, G. (1998). Manager, Committee on Publication, The First Church of Christ, Scientist, Boston, MA.

Magida, A. J. (Ed.). (1996). Christian Science. *How to be a perfect stranger.* Woodstock, NY: Jewish Lights Publishing.

Park Ridge Center for the Study of Health, Faith, and Ethics. (1996). *The Christian Science tradition: Religious beliefs and health care decisions.* Chicago, IL: Park Ridge Center.

Peel, R. (1988). *Health and medicine in the Christian Science tradition.* New York: Crossroad Publishing.

Websites: *www.christianscience.org, www.tfccs.com,* and *www.marybakereddy.org*

Hinduism

Introduction

This information is given as an introduction to a specific religious tradition and is meant to help providers understand similarities and variations among religious practices. Providers are cautioned not to overgeneralize or characterize all members of a religious group as alike. In fact, a person's spiritual and religious profile is unique and can be determined only when trust has been established and open-ended assessment questions have been asked.

The provider is encouraged to inquire about the family's spiritual needs near the end of an initial interview. Perhaps the topic can be introduced by saying: "We know that illness can be very stressful. Many families find their faith or spiritual beliefs a source of strength or comfort during a hospital stay. I'm wondering if your spirituality or religion is important to you?" If the patient or family says "yes," these questions follow naturally:*

"Do you follow a particular religious tradition or spiritual path?" If the answer is yes, "Would you like a visit from your own clergy or a hospital chaplain during your stay?" If the answer is yes, "Would you like to include that person in the conversation when it comes time to make an important treatment decision?"

Some other possible questions include the following:

- "Are there religious customs or spiritual practices that are important to you, but likely to be disrupted during this hospital stay or illness?"

- "Are there ways that we can help you maintain your spiritual strength or routine during this stay (for example, worship opportunities, medals, devotional materials, kosher meals, Sabbath candles, communion, baptism, prayer rug, and so forth)?"

- "How does your faith influence the way you think about this illness?"

When making an assessment, additional factors to consider include age, gender, ethnic group, developmental stage, family structure, faith community, life experiences, psychosocial history, and individual characteristics. Providers should consult the hospital chaplain for assistance with an assessment.

The following information is provided on Hindu practices and traditions.

---

* These questions were adapted from L. Carpenito, *Nursing Diagnosis: Application to Clinical Practice* (7th ed.). New York: Lippincott Williams & Wilkins, 1997.

In Brief

- Hinduism may be the world's oldest religion, dating back to 1,000 B.C. It originated in Southern Asia in what are now the countries of India, Pakistan, Nepal, and Sri Lanka.

- About 20 percent of Indians practice a faith other than Hinduism, so the health care provider must not assume that all Indians are Hindus.

- There are approximately 1.3 million practicing Hindus in North America.

- Hinduism does not have one singular doctrine or founder.

- Sacred texts include the Bhagavad-Gita, Vedas, and Upanishads.

- Hinduism posits that one's purpose or self-realization is achieved through not one but many paths, depending on one's "dharma" or moral duty in life. Dharma can vary with occupation or stage of life.

- The tradition honors one god, who is worshipped in different forms. One's ultimate goal of existence in life is to be able to obtain "Nirvana," or oneness with God.

- Hindu worship is typically private and centered around the household altar, the temple, or a pilgrimage to holy sites.

- Hindus believe that living a pure and ethical life that is caring of others determines one's fate in a future life. It is the hope that one will spiritually progress in subsequent reincarnations to union with the holy being. The concept of "Karma" suggests that one's current way of life and actions will affect one's future.

- Many believe that faith and prayer can heal.

Place of Worship

Worship is at the temple and household altar.

Clergy

Priests, who are called "Swamiji" (pronounced "Swameejee") lead the worship.

Holy Days

Hindus celebrate many holidays, and the significance varies depending on where in South Asia the family comes from. Many Hindus celebrate the following holidays, with the exact dates varying year to year: "Diwali" (late fall)—Festival of Light, a time of gift giving and family festivity; "Shivra Ratri" (late winter)—all night worship; "Duhsehra" or "Durga Puja" (early autumn); "Rama Navami" (spring)—Festival of Colors, and Krishna's birthday (late summer).

Religious Observance in the Hospital Setting

Worship   There are many forms of Hindu devotions, including meditation using a "mantra" (the repetition of certain words or sounds), reverence of deity images, the use of holy water from the Ganges river in India, yoga, physical gestures, and offerings of food ("prasad") or flowers.

Most Hindu worship takes place in the home or the temple. In the hospital setting, families may wish to display a picture of a deity or to meditate.

Dietary Needs   Many, but not all, Hindus are vegetarians. Many do not eat beef, white meats, or eggs, believing that they are sacred. Many of the Hindu holy days involve fasting or abstinence from eating grains.

Care of the Sick   *Pastoral Care.* Hindus are generally receptive to a visit from the hospital chaplain. They do not expect a visit from Hindu clergy during a hospital stay.

Treatment. Blood products, organ donations, and most medications are permitted. Many Hindus eat with their right hand and reserve the left hand for toileting and washing. Therefore, they may prefer the right hand for placement of an IV.

Special Concerns   *Birth.* Ceremonies for the naming of infants vary widely, depending on geographic region, and typically take place outside the hospital. A Hindu child may receive many names. The last name is most appropriate for the medical record. Most Hindus do not circumcise male infants. Circumcision has a strong historical reference for the Hindu population, and providers should use sensitivity when offering this option.

Modesty. Females should be examined by females and males by males, whenever possible. Hindus may be very uncomfortable with the hospital gowns that we offer and may prefer clothing from home. This alternative should be explored with the family.

Surgery. Many Hindus may consult an astrological chart when choosing optimum dates for surgery.

Death. Hindus believe that although the physical body dies, the soul of a person has no beginning or end ("Samsara"). Death marks a passage, rather than the end of life. At death, the soul may be reborn into another living being. The nature of subsequent rebirth is a consequence of actions taken in this life.

The family may wish to keep vigil at the bedside and play recordings of sacred Indian music to help the patient detach from pain or other worldly things. While the burning of incense is not permitted in the hospital, special arrangements may be made for the use of incense in the hospital chapel or prayer room. The ashes from the incense are often placed on the forehead of the patient, as a blessing.

Hindu clergy are not usually requested; if present, clergy may tie sacred threads around the wrists or neck of the body. Providers should not remove these threads.

After death, the family may wish to place drops of holy water and basil leaves in the mouth of the deceased, as well as wash or dress the body. The clinician should wear disposable gloves to show respect in closing the eyes and wrapping the body. The deceased's arms should be straightened.

Hindus may prefer to use a funeral home that is familiar with traditional rituals and practices. Hindus new to the United States may appreciate assistance in making arrangements. Consultation with the hospital chaplain may be helpful.

Cremation is preferred, usually within twenty-four hours of death. Survivors may choose to fast until the cremation takes place. If so, families may appreciate advocacy to ensure prompt cremation. Family members sometimes choose to delay the cremation until the arrival of extended family. In either case, embalming is not customary. The remains are usually scattered in the Ganges or another body of water.

A bereavement ceremony to assist the well-being of the soul takes place in the home between ten and thirty days after death, often on the thirteenth day. The first-year anniversary and subsequent anniversaries of death are very important to surviving family members and involve sacred religious rites.

Autopsy. Autopsy is permissible.

References

Desai, P. (1990). *Health and medicine in the Hindu tradition.* New York: Crossroad Publishing.

Kirkwood, N. (1995). *Hospital handbook on multiculturalism and religion.* Harrisburg, PA: Morehouse.

Lipson, J. G., Dibble, S. L., & Minarik, P. A. (Eds.). (1997). Hinduism. *Culture and nursing care: A pocket guide.* San Francisco: University of California San Francisco Nursing Press.

Sullivan, E. (1989). *Healing and restoring: Health and medicine in the world's religious traditions.* New York: Macmillan.

Websites: *www.hindunet.org* and *www.hindu.org*

Islam (the Faith of Muslims)

Introduction

This information is given as an introduction to a specific religious tradition and is meant to help providers understand similarities and variations among religious practices. Providers are cautioned not to overgeneralize or characterize all members of a religious group as alike. In fact, a person's spiritual and religious profile is unique and can be determined only when trust has been established and open-ended assessment questions have been asked.

The provider is encouraged to inquire about the family's spiritual needs near the end of an initial interview. Perhaps the topic can be introduced by saying: "We know that illness can be very stressful. Many families find their faith or spiritual beliefs a source of strength or comfort during a hospital stay. I'm wondering if your spirituality or religion is important to you?" If the patient or family says "yes," these questions follow naturally:*

"Do you follow a particular religious tradition or spiritual path?" If the answer is yes, "Would you like a visit from your own clergy or a hospital chaplain during your stay?" If the answer is yes, "Would you like to include that person in the conversation when it comes time to make an important treatment decision?"

Some other possible questions include the following:

- "Are there religious customs or spiritual practices that are important to you, but likely to be disrupted during this hospital stay or illness?"

- "Are there ways that we can help you maintain your spiritual strength or routine during this stay (for example, worship opportunities, medals, devotional materials, kosher meals, Sabbath candles, communion, baptism, prayer rug, and so forth)?"

- "How does your faith influence the way you think about this illness?"

When making an assessment, additional factors to consider include age, gender, ethnic group, developmental stage, family structure, faith community, life experiences, psychosocial history, and individual characteristics. Providers should consult the hospital chaplain for assistance with an assessment.

---

* These questions were adapted from L. Carpenito, *Nursing Diagnosis: Application to Clinical Practice* (7th ed.). New York: Lippincott Williams & Wilkins, 1997.

The following information is about Muslim practices and traditions.

In Brief

- Islam is the fastest growing religion in America.
- Muslims are ethnically diverse. There are Muslim communities in nearly every country in the world.
- In the Islamic faith, most matters of everyday life are guided by religious instruction. Islam, like Christianity and Judaism, affirms the oneness of God ("Allah").
- Mohammed is revered as the greatest and final prophet.
- The Koran ("Quran") is the most holy book of Islam.

Place of Worship

A mosque is the main place of worship for Muslims.

Clergy

Muslim clergy are called "imam."

Holy Days

Muslims pray five times a day—at dawn, sunrise, noon, afternoon, sunset, and night. There is a communal gathering for prayers on Friday at midday. Special holy days include Ramadan (the holy month of fasting), "Eidul-Fitr" (breaking the fast at the close of Ramadan), and "Eidul Adha" (the feast of sacrifice).

Religious Observance in the Hospital Setting

Worship   Most Muslims pray facing east (toward the sacred house in Mecca). It is customary to pray on the floor, using a prayer rug. Prayers take only a matter of minutes, and families may wish to pray in their room rather than go to the hospital chapel. Nurses may offer a clean bed sheet as a prayer rug and facilitate privacy by putting a sign on the door during prayer times. Preparation for worship includes meticulous washing of the face, feet to ankles, and hands to elbows.

Because Muslims use the right hand for washing and other bodily functions, it would be appropriate to place an IV in the left hand.

It is common for Muslims to say "In the name of Allah the compassionate, the merciful" before all meaningful activities in the day, including a medical or nursing procedure.

Dietary Needs   Consumption of pork and alcohol are prohibited. All other meats must be slaughtered in a ritual way, called "halal." Kosher food meets Muslim requirements. Kosher meals can often be ordered for patients and families from the hospital cafeteria. Muslim families often prefer to bring prepared food from home and need a place to refrigerate it.

The twenty-nine-day or thirty-day period of Ramadan, an Islamic holiday, begins in either December or January, depending on the Islamic lunar calendar. Neither food nor drink is to pass between the lips between dawn and sunset. Young children and the sick are exempt, but may need the encouragement of the imam to eat.

Care of the Sick   *Pastoral Care.* An imam may visit the patient and family in the hospital. The imam provides spiritual and emotional support as well as reads passages from the Koran. Muslim families typically consult with an imam about complex medical or ethical decisions.

Treatment. Muslims often believe that Allah has determined everything that happens in a person's life, including the place and time of death. Therefore, complaints about life events, feelings of powerlessness, or anger are not usually expressed among Muslims.

Trust in Allah is the primary coping mechanism for Muslims. Although they view the medical and nursing team as skilled technicians and have high regard for science, all outcomes from death to recovery are seen as Allah's doing.

Decisions regarding medical care at the end of life are usually made on a case-by-case basis in consultation with an imam, and optimally with the second opinion of a Muslim physician. Although it may be a challenge to locate a Muslim physician within the appropriate specialty, it is greatly appreciated by the families. The imam from the nearest mosque can be a resource for health care providers.

Special Concerns   *Decision Making.* The father is usually a Muslim family's public spokesperson and the one who signs consent forms. Mothers are very involved in private consultations between parents, especially when matters relate to children. Although both parents should be included in family conferences, the mother will probably choose to be silent in that setting.

Muslim families may ask fewer questions of staff than others; asking questions is considered a sign of mistrust.

Anxiety. Muslims may have come from parts of the world in which they did not have freedom of religion or speech. It is common for Muslims to be afraid that they will be harmed by others because of their religion.

They may be afraid to disclose their religious preference. A visit from an imam or a Muslim chaplain can often reassure families in the hospital setting.

Nudity. Modesty is very important to Muslims. After puberty, Muslim women are usually expected to cover their whole body with the exception of parts of the face and the hands. Some might choose to cover their faces also. Facial coverings are worn only in the presence of nonimmediate male relatives or male strangers. For this reason, families may prefer a private hospital room. Men are traditionally covered from waist to knee, even in front of other men. Females should be examined by females and males by males, whenever possible. Care providers should knock before entering a hospital room, allowing time for the women to cover themselves.

Muslims may be very uncomfortable with the hospital gowns that are offered and may prefer clothing from home. This alternative should be explored with the family.

Gender. In the pediatric setting where a parent sleeps at the child's bedside, a private room is preferred. Religious law prohibits a married woman from sleeping in the same room as a man who is not her husband.

Death. The family of a dying Muslim may ask that the patient face east, with his or her head elevated. At the time of death, the Muslim call to prayer is recited by friends, and a chapter of the Koran is read aloud. Copies of the Koran should be made available through the hospital chaplain. An imam is not customarily present at the time of death, but will come if asked.

Postmortem Care. Health care providers should speak with the family or the Muslim chaplain before giving postmortem care. Many may prefer that another Muslim of the same sex prepare the body. If no Muslim is present, a non-Muslim should use gloves when touching the body. The body should be draped to ensure privacy at all times. Washing will be done in a ritual way at the funeral home. When doing the postmortem care, the head should be turned to the right, and the arms laid by the patient's side. The patient's hair should not be cut.

Autopsy. The body is considered sacred; therefore, autopsies are forbidden except in cases of compelling legal or medical reasons. If an autopsy must be done, it should be as non-invasive and minimally disfiguring as possible (for example, a tissue biopsy), and all body parts and fluids should be returned to the body for burial. Special funeral homes familiar with Muslim customs are preferred.

Burial Customs. Burial is performed as soon as possible, as embalming is not customary. Cremation is forbidden.

Organ Transplantation. There are no restrictions on organ transplantation, as long as organs are donated and received as gifts. Organs may not be purchased or sold.

References

Websites: *www.fas.harvard.edu/~pluralsm, www.islamworld.net/wings.buffalo. edu/sa/muslim/isl/isl.html,   www.bev.net/community/sedki/IslamicCenter. html* and *www.beconvinced.com*

Jehovah's Witness

Introduction

This information is given as an introduction to a specific religious tradition and is meant to help providers understand similarities and variations among religious practices. Providers are cautioned not to overgeneralize or characterize all members of a religious group as alike. In fact, a person's spiritual and religious profile is unique and can be determined only when trust has been established and open-ended assessment questions have been asked.

The provider is encouraged to inquire about the family's spiritual needs near the end of an initial interview. Perhaps the topic can be introduced by saying: "We know that illness can be very stressful. Many families find their faith or spiritual beliefs a source of strength or comfort during a hospital stay. I'm wondering if your spirituality or religion is important to you?" If the patient or family says "yes," these questions follow naturally:*

"Do you follow a particular religious tradition or spiritual path?" If the answer is yes, "Would you like a visit from your own clergy or a hospital chaplain during your stay?" If the answer is yes, "Would you like to include that person in the conversation when it comes time to make an important treatment decision?"

Some other possible questions include the following:

- "Are there religious customs or spiritual practices that are important to you, but likely to be disrupted during this hospital stay or illness?"

- "Are there ways that we can help you maintain your spiritual strength or routine during this stay (for example, worship opportunities, medals, devotional materials, kosher meals, Sabbath candles, communion, baptism, prayer rug, and so forth)?"

- "How does your faith influence the way you think about this illness?"

When making an assessment, additional factors to consider include age, gender, ethnic group, developmental stage, family structure, faith community, life experiences, psychosocial history, and individual characteristics. Providers should consult the hospital chaplain for assistance with an assessment.

---

* These questions were adapted from L. Carpenito, *Nursing Diagnosis: Application to Clinical Practice* (7th ed.). New York: Lippincott Williams & Wilkins, 1997.

The following information is about Jehovah's Witnesses, their practices and traditions.

In Brief

- One of the newest Protestant denominations, Jehovah's Witness was founded in the late 1800s.

- There are now approximately 976,000 Jehovah's Witnesses in the United States and about 5,500,000 worldwide.

- Jehovah's Witnesses use "Jehovah" as their sole name for God. They look forward to an imminent transformation of the world in which Jesus will rule, all wickedness will be eliminated, and the dead will be resurrected to life.

- Jehovah's Witnesses base their beliefs on a literal interpretation of the Bible (Hebrew scriptures and Christian Greek scriptures). Scriptures are used as a guide for all aspects of life, including medical care.

Place of Worship

Local worship centers called Kingdom Hall are used.

Clergy

There are no clergy. Each congregation is supervised by elders, who are the primary teachers, preachers, and hospital visitors.

Holy Days

Most Witnesses do not celebrate birthdays, Christmas, Lent, Easter, or national holidays. Sunday is the usual day of rest and worship.

Religious Observance in the Hospital Setting

Worship

Bedside prayer in the company of a visiting elder is greatly appreciated. Jehovah's Witnesses often appreciate pre-operative prayer. The Protestant chaplain can arrange for a visit from an elder.

Dietary Needs   The scriptures do not state any dietary restrictions.

Care of the Sick   *Choice of Hospital and Physician.* Jehovah's Witnesses generally have a very high regard for medicine and health care professionals. Because Witnesses have strong religious concerns about use of blood products and transfusions, they place high value on family-to-physician communication. Witnesses typically seek specialists whose clinical excellence includes minimization of blood loss and sensitivity to spiritual concerns.

Hospital Liaison Committee. Jehovah's Witnesses have established hospital liaison committees in most cities to provide families with a referral network of physicians and hospitals that have demonstrated sensitivity to the concerns of Jehovah's Witnesses. Families wishing to speak with the Committee may contact the Protestant chaplain or call the national headquarters at (718) 625-3600.

Special Concerns   *Blood Transfusions and Blood Products.* Witnesses will refuse transfusion of whole blood, packed red cells, white blood cells, plasma, and platelets. Pre-operative banking of one's own blood for subsequent transfusion is also prohibited. The prohibition is based on three biblical passages (Genesis 9:3,4; Leviticus 17:10; and Acts 15:28–29), which prohibit the consumption of blood. Jehovah's Witnesses interpret the scriptures to instruct that one cannot take blood into the body by eating and liken transfusion to other forms of consumption.

Many Witnesses will accept albumin, immune globulins, hemophiliac preparations, nonblood volume expanders (including crystalloids, dextrans, and nonblood colloids or oxygen carrying blood substitutes), and pre-operative erythropoietin. They will also accept greater than normal degrees of anemia. These options should be discussed explicitly with the patient and/or legal guardian.

Therapies to reduce blood loss, such as intraoperative blood salvage, acute interoperative hemodilution, laser surgery, coagulating devices, minimum blood draws, and pulse oximeters are encouraged. Cardiac bypass and dialysis are permitted when nonblood products can be used to prime the equipment and the extracorporeal circuit is uninterrupted.

Right to Refuse Blood Products. Jehovah's Witnesses believe the competent patient has the right to refuse blood transfusions and blood products based on the principal of autonomy and freedom of religion. The courts have upheld the competent adult's right to refuse blood transfusion unless the adult is pregnant or there are dependent minor children.

The courts have consistently held that Witnesses cannot refuse medically indicated transfusions for their children, especially when a child's life is in danger. Legal consultation should be sought from the hospital's legal office in such situations.

In most cases, it is productive to anticipate problems by proactively exploring the wishes of Witnesses. Families may wish a second opinion, especially from a physician who has been identified by the Hospital Liaison

Committee. Physicians can consult with the blood bank regarding use of erythropoietin in the weeks prior to surgery.

If a court order is sought, it is important that the parents be informed and be offered the opportunity to articulate their beliefs to the judge with a spiritual advocate present, if desired. The Protestant chaplain can serve in that role or locate a member of the Hospital Liaison Committee at the family's request.

Pastoral Consultation on Refusal of Blood Products. Many Witnesses believe that violating the divine rule about blood will compromise their relationship with God, imperil their chance for eternal life, and create tensions within their congregation. Others believe that one's spiritual integrity is maintained if the transfusion takes place without one's consent (for example, by court order or permission of a parent who is not a Witness). In either case, the patient and family are at risk for spiritual distress, and the services of the Protestant chaplain should be offered.

Abortion. Abortion is not permitted, even when birth defects are diagnosed. If the mother's life is in danger, whether to have an abortion is the parents' decision.

Birth. Witnesses do not practice baptism.

Death. A family might wish the emotional support and prayers of an elder and readings from the scriptures. There are no last rites. Death is understood to be a deep sleep until the time when Jehovah transforms the world, when the dead will be given new life.

Witnesses believe that when death is clearly imminent and unavoidable, extraordinary means of care and resuscitation may be foregone. Any active measures to hasten death, as in active euthanasia, are forbidden.

Organ Transplantation. No scriptural instruction bears on the topic, so Witnesses may decide on an individual basis.

Autopsy. Witnesses will honor legal requirements for an autopsy, but generally decline optional postmortem examination. Either burial or cremation is permissible.

References

Park Ridge Center for the Study of Health, Faith, and Ethics. (1995). *The Jehovah's Witness tradition: Religious beliefs and health care decisions.* Chicago, IL: Park Ridge Center.

Watchtower Bible and Tract Society (1992). *Family care and medical management for Jehovah's Witnesses.* New York: Watchtower.

Websites: *www.harvard.edu/~pluralsm,*   *www.watchtower.org,*   and *www.noblood.com.*

Judaism

Introduction

This information is given as an introduction to a specific religious tradition and is meant to help providers understand similarities and variations among religious practices. Providers are cautioned not to overgeneralize or characterize all members of a religious group as alike. In fact, a person's spiritual and religious profile is unique and can be determined only when trust has been established and open-ended assessment questions have been asked.

The provider is encouraged to inquire about the family's spiritual needs near the end of an initial interview. Perhaps the topic can be introduced by saying: "We know that illness can be very stressful. Many families find their faith or spiritual beliefs a source of strength or comfort during a hospital stay. I'm wondering if your spirituality or religion is important to you?" If the patient or family says "yes," these questions follow naturally:*

"Do you follow a particular religious tradition or spiritual path?" If the answer is yes, "Would you like a visit from your own clergy or a hospital chaplain during your stay?" If the answer is yes, "Would you like to include that person in the conversation when it comes time to make an important treatment decision?"

Some other possible questions include the following:

- "Are there religious customs or spiritual practices that are important to you, but likely to be disrupted during this hospital stay or illness?"

- "Are there ways that we can help you maintain your spiritual strength or routine during this stay (for example, worship opportunities, medals, devotional materials, kosher meals, Sabbath candles, communion, baptism, prayer rug, and so forth)?"

- "How does your faith influence the way you think about this illness?"

When making an assessment, additional factors to consider include age, gender, ethnic group, developmental stage, family structure, faith community, life experiences, psychosocial history, and individual characteristics. Providers should consult the hospital chaplain for assistance with an assessment.

---

* These questions were adapted from L. Carpenito, *Nursing Diagnosis: Application to Clinical Practice* (7th ed.). New York: Lippincott Williams & Wilkins, 1997.

The following information is about Jewish practices and traditions.

In Brief

- Judaism includes religious beliefs and rituals as well as a code of ethical behavior. It remembers the rich history of the Jewish people in its celebrations. Its adherents include people of every race and most nations in the world.

- There are four major Jewish communities in America: Reform, Reconstructionist, Conservative, and Orthodox. There are several other branches of Orthodox Judaism, such as "Hasidism."

- The foundations of Judaism are the Torah (the first five books of the Bible, which recount God's covenant with Abraham and his descendants), and the Talmud (which interprets the Torah).

Place of Worship

Worship is held in a synagogue or temple.

Clergy

Rabbis serve Jewish needs.

Holy Days

The Sabbath ("shabbat" or "shabbos") begins on Friday at sundown and continues to Saturday sundown. Families usually begin the Sabbath by lighting candles and saying a prayer with their mother and other family members. Electric candles may be obtained from the chaplain for the hospital setting.

For the most observant, religious law prohibits riding in a car, smoking, cooking, writing, and handling money on the Sabbath. Use of electricity (such as television, telephone, electric bed, elevator, and so forth) is also forbidden on the Sabbath for those that are most observant. Non-essential tests, written consent, and patient discharges should be avoided on the Sabbath. Lighting needed during the twenty-four hours can be turned on before the Sabbath begins. Sensitivity to the family's obligation to climb stairs in lieu of elevators and discomfort with electrically powered doors, beds, and call bells would be appreciated. The Jewish chaplain can provide information about a Sabbath route that provides electric-free access into and around the hospital.

For all Jews, Sabbath restrictions are canceled in order to save a life. It is wise to anticipate a plan for communicating with a family in the event of a true medical emergency. Offering a beeper or telephone code may be acceptable if agreed to be for emergency use only.

Passover (the celebration of freedom from slavery in Egypt) is held in early spring, "Rosh Ha Shanah" (New Year celebration) is held in the fall, "Yom Kippur" (day of atonement) is in the fall, "Sukkot" (the feast of booths) is in fall, "Shavuot" (the festival of weeks) is in late spring. All are included in Sabbath rules. "Chanukah" (Festival of Lights) in December and "Purim" (in spring) have no such restrictions.

Religious Observance in the Hospital Setting

Worship   Traditional Jews pray three times a day (morning, afternoon, and evening). For morning prayers, people might wear a prayer shawl and "tefillin" (black boxes with leather straps tied to the forehead and left arm). These boxes contain a prayer affirming God's oneness. Privacy for prayer is very important and should be afforded families, even in the busy hospital setting. Orthodox Jews will avoid praying in a room in which the patient expels body fluids. A rabbi is not needed to lead in prayer.

Dietary Needs   For Orthodox and some Conservative Jews, there is no mixing of meat with dairy at a meal. There are separate cooking utensils for meat and dairy. Food prepared according to these strict guidelines is called "kosher." All meat must be slaughtered in a special manner, and no shellfish or unkosher meat is eaten.

Kosher foods are often available in the hospital kitchen and can be ordered for the patient as well as the family through the dietary department. Staff may wish to provide space for refrigeration of kosher foods prepared at home.

During Yom Kippur in the fall, a twenty-four-hour fast is observed. During Sukkot, an eight-day harvest festival in October, families usually eat outside in a special booth built for this purpose. The chaplain may wish to provide such a booth at the hospital for observant families and staff or refer them to one near the hospital. During Passover in April, no leavened products are eaten, and kosher rules are more stringent. During Passover, the Jewish family often gathers for a ritual meal called a "seder." The hospital chaplain may wish to sponsor a seder in the hospital setting for patients and their families. A twenty-four-hour fast day, "Tisha b'av," occurs in the summer.

Care of the Sick   *Pastoral Care.* It is a "mitzvah" (obligation of all Jews) to visit the sick. Jews will expect a visit from friends and family as well as their rabbi. The rabbi will offer support and usually a Hebrew prayer for one's health. One's own rabbi usually visits, although the hospital chaplain is always welcome.

A rabbi is typically consulted for guidance in complex medical or ethical decisions.

Special Concerns   *Birth.* For most Jews, a baby boy is not named until the eighth day of life, when the ritual circumcision is done. A specially trained person ("Mohel") performs circumcision in a ceremony at home. Circumcision may be postponed if the baby is ill. In such a situation, the reassurance of the rabbi may be helpful.

A baby girl is usually officially named during the reading of the Torah at the synagogue. Providers may care for a child who has not yet been named and should not assume that the lack of a name is indicative of poor parental bonding.

Gender. An Orthodox or Hassidic Jewish man will not touch any women other than his wife, daughter, and mother. When greeting an Orthodox or Hassidic male, female providers should offer a nod instead of a handshake. Orthodox or Hassidic women will prefer to be cared for by women, and men by men. In the pediatric setting where a parent sleeps at the child's bedside, a private room is preferred. Religious law prohibits a married woman from sleeping in the same room with a man who is not her husband.

Head Covering. Orthodox and Conservative Hassidic men wear a head covering at all times. Women cover their hair after marriage. Some Orthodox women wear head coverings or wigs as a sign of their piety. Sterile hair coverings should be provided for Orthodox adults prior to surgery.

Discharge. Patients who are discharged on the Sabbath cannot use the telephone to call a family member, nor use cars, taxis, or public transportation. Walking home is permitted. Facilitating discharge before noon on a Friday or after sundown on Saturday is appreciated.

Death. Judaism defines death as occurring when respiration and circulation are irreversibly stopped. Brain death is not generally acknowledged among the most Orthodox and is a source of debate among Conservatives.

Euthanasia and withdrawal of care that hastens death are strictly forbidden. In some cases, extraordinary care may be withheld. There are precise rabbinical guidelines called "Responsa" for such situations, and consultation with the Rabbi about such matters is often sought by the family.

At the time of death, the family may wish to gather at the bedside, read psalms, and recite the "vidui" (last prayer of confession). There are no last rites. It is not customary for a rabbi to be present at the time of death, although one may be requested. Jews do not make funeral arrangements on the Sabbath or major holidays.

Postmortem Care. Postmortem care is very important to observant Jews. Medical personnel should consult the family before washing the body. The nurse should wear gloves when providing routine care of the body. The arms of the deceased are not crossed in postmortem care. Any clothing, dressings, or medical equipment with the patient's blood must be buried with the patient.

The Jewish community may use designated individuals to wash the body at a later time and prefer funeral homes that are familiar with Jewish faith and ritual.

In the Jewish tradition, the body may not be left alone until the burial. Family may wish to station someone outside the morgue to sit near the body until it is removed from the hospital. Burial should take place within twenty-four hours. Efforts on the part of staff to expedite arrangements are appreciated.

Autopsy. Some Orthodox and Conservative Jews do not approve of autopsy, unless it is required by law or the life of a specific person (for example, other family members in the case of a hereditary illness) can be saved by information from the autopsy.

If an autopsy is done, the more limited the disfigurement, the better (needle biopsy, limited autopsy, or in situ examination are preferred). Some Orthodox and Conservative Jews may request that all body parts and fluids be returned for burial, even when it may limit potential findings. Some Orthodox families may request that their rabbi be present to observe the autopsy.

Burial Customs. Cremation is forbidden. Burial is required to be done as soon as possible. Embalming is not permitted unless legally required.

A mourning period follows the funeral for the immediate family ("Shiva"). Friends and hospital staff who have come to know the family well are welcome to visit the home during the mourning period. Providers unfamiliar with the visiting customs should consult the Jewish chaplain.

It is customary to make charitable contributions rather than send flowers.

References

Magida, A. J. (Ed.). (1996). Judaism. *How to be a perfect stranger.* Woodstock, NY: Jewish Lights Publishing.

Park Ridge Center for the Study of Health, Faith, and Ethics. (1996). *The Jewish tradition: Religious beliefs and health care decisions.* Chicago, IL: Park Ridge Center.

Websites: *www.jewfaq.org,*   *http://shamash.org/trb/judaism.html*   and *www.jewishhealth.com*

Eastern Orthodox

Introduction

This information is given as an introduction to a specific religious tradition and is meant to help providers understand similarities and variations among religious practices. Providers are cautioned not to overgeneralize or characterize all members of a religious group as alike. In fact, a person's spiritual and religious profile is unique and can be determined only when trust has been established and open-ended assessment questions have been asked.

The provider is encouraged to inquire about the family's spiritual needs near the end of an initial interview. Perhaps the topic can be introduced by saying: "We know that illness can be very stressful. Many families find their faith or spiritual beliefs a source of strength or comfort during a hospital stay. I'm wondering if your spirituality or religion is important to you?" If the patient or family says "yes," these questions follow naturally:*

"Do you follow a particular religious tradition or spiritual path?" If the answer is yes, "Would you like a visit from your own clergy or a hospital chaplain during your stay?" If the answer is yes, "Would you like to include that person in the conversation when it comes time to make an important treatment decision?"

Some other possible questions include the following:

- "Are there religious customs or spiritual practices that are important to you, but likely to be disrupted during this hospital stay or illness?"

- "Are there ways that we can help you maintain your spiritual strength or routine during this stay (for example, worship opportunities, medals, devotional materials, kosher meals, Sabbath candles, communion, baptism, prayer rug, and so forth)?"

- "How does your faith influence the way you think about this illness?"

When making an assessment, additional factors to consider include age, gender, ethnic group, developmental stage, family structure, faith community, life experiences, psychosocial history, and individual characteristics. Providers should consult the hospital chaplain for assistance with an assessment.

---

* These questions were adapted from L. Carpenito, *Nursing Diagnosis: Application to Clinical Practice* (7th ed.). New York: Lippincott Williams & Wilkins, 1997.

The following information is provided about Orthodox practices and traditions.

In Brief

- The Christian church was established early in the 1st Century. Gradually the Eastern and Western churches grew apart, following disagreements over their beliefs. The Western church became known as the Roman Catholic Church. It is based in Rome under the direction of the Pope. The Eastern church became known as the Orthodox church, based in Istanbul under the direction of the Ecumenical Patriarch of Constantinople.

- There are many Orthodox churches in America. The Greek Orthodox Church is the largest, with an estimated membership of 1.5 million. The Russian Orthodox Church (Orthodox Church in America) and the Albanian, Armenian, Antiochian, Ethiopian, Romanian, Serbian, Syrian, and Ukrainian churches have smaller memberships.

- In general, Orthodox churches share the same faith beliefs, but have diverse cultural influences and languages associated with their specific geographic areas of origin.

- The Bible is the guiding text, which is complemented by a very rich and important oral tradition.

- The Greek Orthodox Church is known for its tradition in worship and liturgy, which centers on holy sacraments. Icons (two-dimensional images of the saints, as well as of Biblical personalities or events), incense, and the Greek language enrich the worship experience.

Place of Worship

Church on Sunday mornings and on major feast days.

Clergy

There are three orders of clergy: deacons, priests or presbyters, who are addressed as "Father," and bishops. All are male. Both deacons and priests may marry.

Holy Days

Christmas, Epiphany (January 6), Easter or "Pascha," and Pentecost (seventh Sunday after Easter). The date for the Greek Orthodox Easter may differ from the Catholic or Protestant observance.

Religious Observance in the Hospital Setting

Worship   Many Greek Orthodox persons will bring a favorite icon to facilitate their prayers. Such objects are often unique family heirlooms and care should be taken with them.

The priest is expected to visit on behalf of the church community. A blessing and Holy Communion, offered by the priest, are highly valued before surgery.

Communion should be scheduled the day before surgery, because a patient cannot receive food the morning of surgery. Providers should refer communion requests to the family's clergy or the hospital chaplain's office.

In some cases, Orthodox persons may wish to have the opportunity for confession. An Orthodox priest should be called, and the opportunity for complete privacy should be provided.

Dietary Needs   Observant adults in the Greek Orthodox Church refrain from eating meat and dairy products on most Wednesdays, Fridays, and selected holy days. Seasons for fasting include forty days prior to Christmas and forty-nine days prior to Easter. Seriously ill patients are excluded from this dietary obligation.

Care of the Sick   *Pastoral Care.* It is customary for the priest to visit the mother and child on the day after birth to offer prayers for postpartum healing and protection.

In the event that the child's life is in danger, providers should ask the family about baptism. A simple baptism service can be celebrated in the hospital with the family's clergy, or a chaplain can be called in the event of a life-threatening emergency.

Special Concerns   *Euthanasia.* The Greek Orthodox tradition is against euthanasia, although there is no obligation to prolong life when it is clear that death is imminent and inevitable.

Death. When a person nears death, providers should arrange to call the priest of the family's church. If the family does not have a local clergy member, the hospital chaplain may assist in contacting an Orthodox priest through the local diocese. If the patient is awake, Holy Communion should be offered to the dying patient. The Orthodox priest may also anoint the patient on the forehead, cheeks, chest, and hands with holy oil in a ritual of spiritual and bodily healing known as the Sacrament of the Holy Unction. There are no "Last Rites" in the Greek Orthodox Church.

If the patient has died, the priest will read special prayers for the dead and provide support to the bereaved.

Family members may prefer to use a funeral home that is familiar with the Greek Orthodox traditions. For example, when Greek Orthodox children die, great care is taken in the selection of burial clothing. It is customary to dress the child in white as if a bride or groom of Christ.

Cremation is forbidden. Those wishing a funeral in the church will choose burial.

Autopsy. Greek Orthodox persons usually decline autopsies, although they are permitted if there are compelling medical reasons for one. Orthodox persons may prefer that all tissues and organs be returned to the body for burial (Harakas, 1990).

Organ Donation. The Greek Orthodox have no official position regarding organ donation. Many view donation as an act of love and generosity, while others have religious concerns about the integrity of the body. Providers should offer the family the opportunity to consult with an Orthodox priest.

Abortion. The Greek Orthodox Church officially opposes all forms of abortion, even in the event of diagnosed anomalies or illness (Harakas, 1990). Exceptions to this principle may be considered in cases of thalassemia (a hereditary, chronic anemia affecting families of Mediterranean descent) or when the life of the mother is endangered. In such cases, providers should encourage the family to consult with an Orthodox priest.

Contraception. "The Greek Orthodox Church takes no official position on contraception. Generally speaking, contraception within the context of marriage is accepted when it facilitates the spacing of children and the health of the marital relationship" (Harakas, 1990).

Suicide. The taking of one's own life is considered comparable to the taking of another's; it is considered a grave sin. The Greek Orthodox Church will provide a funeral to a suicide victim if, in the opinion of a physician, the person was mentally ill and incapable of making a reasoned decision.

References

Greek Orthodox Archdiocese of America yearbook. (1998). New York: Delta Printing.

Harakas, S. (1990). *Health and medicine in the Eastern Orthodox tradition.* New York: Crossroad Publishing.

Magida, A. J. (Ed.). (1996). Greek Orthodox. *How to be a perfect stranger.* Woodstock, NY: Jewish Lights Publishing.

Websites: *www.fas.harvard.edu/~pluralsm,   www.christianity.net,   www.webcom.com/~ninnet/xianres.html* and *www.orthodox.org*

Protestantism (Christian)

Introduction

This information is given as an introduction to a specific religious tradition and is meant to help providers understand similarities and variations among religious practices. Providers are cautioned not to overgeneralize or characterize all members of a religious group as alike. In fact, a person's spiritual and religious profile is unique and can be determined only when trust has been established and open-ended assessment questions have been asked.

The provider is encouraged to inquire about the family's spiritual needs near the end of an initial interview. Perhaps the topic can be introduced by saying: "We know that illness can be very stressful. Many families find their faith or spiritual beliefs a source of strength or comfort during a hospital stay. I'm wondering if your spirituality or religion is important to you?" If the patient or family says "yes," these questions follow naturally:*

"Do you follow a particular religious tradition or spiritual path?" If the answer is yes, "Would you like a visit from your own clergy or a hospital chaplain during your stay?" If the answer is yes, "Would you like to include that person in the conversation when it comes time to make an important treatment decision?"

Some other possible questions include the following:

- "Are there religious customs or spiritual practices that are important to you, but likely to be disrupted during this hospital stay or illness?"

- "Are there ways that we can help you maintain your spiritual strength or routine during this stay (for example, worship opportunities, medals, devotional materials, kosher meals, Sabbath candles, communion, baptism, prayer rug, and so forth)?"

- "How does your faith influence the way you think about this illness?"

When making an assessment, additional factors to consider include age, gender, ethnic group, developmental stage, family structure, faith community, life experiences, psychosocial history, and individual characteristics. Providers should consult the hospital chaplain for assistance with an assessment.

---

* These questions were adapted from L. Carpenito, *Nursing Diagnosis: Application to Clinical Practice* (7th ed.). New York: Lippincott Williams & Wilkins, 1997.

The following information is about Protestant practices and traditions.

In Brief

- Protestantism includes a variety of Christian traditions that are not Roman Catholic or Orthodox. Their views and practices differ widely.

- Some Protestant denominations include Assembly of God, Baptist, Christian and Missionary Alliance, Church of the Brethren, Church of Christ, Church of the Nazarene, Congregational, Disciples of Christ, Episcopal, Lutheran, Mennonite, Methodist, Pentecostal, Presbyterian, Reformed, Salvation Army, Seventh Day Adventist, Society of Friends, Unitarian Universalist, United Church of Christ, Wesleyan, and others. Other Christian groups, such as Christian Scientists, Jehovah's Witnesses, and Mormons are covered elsewhere in this chapter, as they have distinctive concerns in the health care setting, although they are in the Protestant tradition and are cared for by Protestant chaplains in most hospitals.

- Protestant Christianity is characterized by a personal relationship with God, study of the Bible by laypersons, freedom of conscience on many matters, and a variety in worship styles.

- Most Protestant churches are autonomous in their operation. Beliefs and practices can vary even within the same denomination.

- The Christian Bible (which includes Hebrew Scriptures and the New Testament) is foundational. Some traditions have an additional holy book.

Place of Worship

Members meet for worship in a church, meeting hall, or meeting house.

Clergy

Not all traditions have clergy. When they do, the clergy is often addressed as "Pastor," "Reverend," or "Elder." The Protestant chaplain in a hospital is usually addressed as "Reverend."

Holy Days

Typically Sunday is the day of worship, although some denominations follow the Jewish tradition of sundown Friday until sundown Saturday; other holy days include Christmas, Ash Wednesday, Maundy Thursday, Good Friday, and Easter.

Religious Observance in the Hospital Setting

Worship   Protestant patients often bring their own Bibles to the hospital and may read them on a daily basis. If they do not have a Bible, the provider may obtain one from the chaplain's office.

Protestants may have their own routine for daily reading and prayer called "devotions." Allowing quiet and uninterrupted time for devotions is appreciated.

Families may prefer their private worship to a chapel service when they are away from their home church.

Persons of the Episcopal and Lutheran traditions may desire communion during their stay. The nurse may contact the Protestant chaplain or church pastor to bring bedside communion.

Dietary Needs   Some religious groups abstain from tobacco, beverages with caffeine, and alcohol. Some are vegetarian. The provider might inquire if there are dietary practices specific to the religious tradition of the patient.

Care of the Sick   *Pastoral Care.* The pastor is expected to visit on behalf of the church community and offer prayer, sacrament, and emotional support. This is true even if the patient is hospitalized out of state. Chaplains may contact the church pastor with the permission of the family. The pastor is often asked to consult in complex medical or ethical decisions.

Prayer. Prayers for the sick are very important to most people of the Protestant faith. Often the pastor or elders in the church will gather at the bedside to pray for the patient. This may be repeated many times. Hymns may be sung. Some traditions anoint the sick with holy oils at this time.

Treatment. Protestants have divergent opinions about withdrawal of life support, euthanasia, abortion, organ transplantation, and blood transfusions.

In general, the most conservative Protestant groups emphasize that God is all-powerful, that all things that happen are planned by God, and that end-of-life decisions are best left to God. Such groups tend to decline abortion, withdrawal of care, and Do Not Resuscitate (DNR). For these groups, organ donation or removal of organs during autopsy is often avoided, as many believe that all body parts need to be buried with the deceased for life after death.

The liberal Protestant traditions allow for individuals to decide such matters on a case-by-case basis, often in consultation with their pastor. Divergence of opinion is commonplace, even within the same family.

Special Concerns   *Blood Transfusions.* Some groups, such as Jehovah's Witnesses, discussed on pages 131 through 134, have specific religious objections to blood products and transfusions. Alternatives to blood transfusions, such as the pre-operative use of erythropoietin, intraoperative blood salvage, and nonblood volume expanders can be explored. Some blood related therapies are optional: albumin, immune globulins, hemophiliac preparations, hemodialysis, and heart bypass. In life-threatening situations, the medical team may seek a court order to transfuse a child against the wishes of the patient or family. Because spiritual distress in the patient and family is a real possibility, the Protestant chaplain should be consulted for follow-up care.

Birth. Some Protestant churches baptize infants. Some baptize only adults when they are old enough to choose a faith tradition. Some churches do not baptize at all.

If a child is critically ill, the nurse may want to ask the family about baptism. If the family wishes to baptize their child in the hospital, the Protestant chaplain can be paged or the church pastor called.

Death. The family usually prefers to be at the bedside of a dying patient and often finds the pastor to be a reassuring companion at such a time. Providers should inquire whether families would like to call their own pastor or the chaplain.

There are no essential end-of-life sacraments, although some Episcopalian, Lutheran, and Pentecostal persons may request anointing. Reading of scripture, bedside prayers that are personalized to the particular situation, and singing are common.

Burial Customs. Funerals, memorial services, and burials are scheduled at the family's convenience, as embalming and/or cremation are common.

Social Services and Discharge Planning. The church may provide meals, transportation, assistance with chores, respite care, and financial assistance to families with illness and should be considered as a valuable resource for family support and discharge planning.

References

Magida, A. J. (Ed.). (1996). Protestantism. *How to be a perfect stranger.* Woodstock, NY: Jewish Lights Publishing.

Park Ridge Center for the Study of Health, Faith, and Ethics. (1996). *The Protestant tradition: Religious beliefs and health care decisions.* Chicago: Park Ridge Center.

Websites: *www.fas.harvard.edu/~pluralsm, www.webcom/~nlnnet/xianres. html,* and *www.christianity.net*

Roman Catholicism

Introduction

This information is given as an introduction to a specific religious tradition and is meant to help providers understand similarities and variations among religious practices. Providers are cautioned not to overgeneralize or characterize all members of a religious group as alike. In fact, a person's spiritual and religious profile is unique and can be determined only when trust has been established and open-ended assessment questions have been asked.

The provider is encouraged to inquire about the family's spiritual needs near the end of an initial interview. Perhaps the topic can be introduced by saying: "We know that illness can be very stressful. Many families find their faith or spiritual beliefs a source of strength or comfort during a hospital stay. I'm wondering if your spirituality or religion is important to you?" If the patient or family says "yes," these questions follow naturally:*

"Do you follow a particular religious tradition or spiritual path?" If the answer is yes, "Would you like a visit from your own clergy or a hospital chaplain during your stay?" If the answer is yes, "Would you like to include that person in the conversation when it comes time to make an important treatment decision?"

Some other possible questions include the following:

- "Are there religious customs or spiritual practices that are important to you, but likely to be disrupted during this hospital stay or illness?"

- "Are there ways that we can help you maintain your spiritual strength or routine during this stay (for example, worship opportunities, medals, devotional materials, kosher meals, Sabbath candles, communion, baptism, prayer rug, and so forth)?"

- "How does your faith influence the way you think about this illness?"

When making an assessment, additional factors to consider include age, gender, ethnic group, developmental stage, family structure, faith community, life experiences, psychosocial history, and individual characteristics. Providers should consult the hospital chaplain for assistance with an assessment.

---

* These questions were adapted from L. Carpenito, *Nursing Diagnosis: Application to Clinical Practice* (7th ed.). New York: Lippincott Williams & Wilkins, 1997.

The following information is about Roman Catholic practices and traditions.

In Brief

- The oldest Christian tradition, the Roman Catholic Church acknowledges the authority of the Pope and the Vatican as its governing body.

- Like all Christians, Roman Catholics believe in the oneness of God, as known in "The Father, the Son (Jesus Christ), and the Holy Spirit."

- The New American Bible or other Catholic translations of Hebrew scriptures and the New Testament are the foundations for worship.

Place of Worship

A Catholic church is the place of worship.

Clergy

Priests (addressed as "Father"), deacons (addressed as "Deacon"), and nuns (addressed as "Sister") lead the church. Catholic hospital chaplains may be any of the above, as well as a lay person.

Holy Days

Every Sunday is considered holy. Special holy days include Christmas, Ash Wednesday, Holy Thursday, Good Friday, and Easter. Additional festival days are celebrated throughout the church year.

Religious Observance in the Hospital Setting

Worship   Sunday worship is called "Mass." Catholics usually attend Mass once a week and on special holy days. A patient or family member may wish to go to Mass when in the hospital setting. In addition to praying to God, Catholics may pray to Mary (the mother of Jesus) as well as the saints, designated holy persons who can spiritually advocate on one's behalf. One common form of prayer is facilitated by a string of beads called a rosary, where each bead is used in a meditative way to recall the life of Christ.

Dietary Needs   Catholics have few special dietary requirements, although they often refrain from eating meat on Fridays in spring, during the penitential season of "Lent" (the forty days before Easter).

Care of the Sick   *Pastoral Care.* Each church parish has a geographic boundary. When someone is hospitalized outside of the parish's geographic boundary, his or her spiritual care is transferred to the hospital chaplain or, in the absence of a chaplain, to the nearest parish.

Prayer. Prayer is highly valued in the hospital setting. Providers should consider the possibility that a prayer (blessing) may be desired preoperatively or before any major procedure, such as a bone marrow transplant. Any Catholic chaplain may provide prayers.

Sacraments. Baptism is an essential sacrament for a Roman Catholic and should be offered whenever a child's life is in danger. It is a one-time sacrament. Any chaplain can baptize in an emergency, and a nurse or parent may do so if a chaplain is not available. The chaplain should be notified when a baptism has taken place so that it can be registered in the local parish and a certificate can be given to the patient.

The deceased are not baptized. Families may request baptism at the time of stillbirth or miscarriage, but typically the chaplain will ritually name the child and offer prayer to commend the child to God's care.

The Sacrament of the Sick is another way that Catholics receive spiritual strength in times of illness. It used to be associated with death ("Last Rites"), but is now offered at any time of sickness. The sacrament includes anointing with oil and prayers. It is not customary for children under the age of seven, but many families may request it for their children near the time of death. The Sacrament of the Sick can only be administered by a priest.

The Sacrament of Reconciliation involves confessing one's sins in order to experience God's love and forgiveness. Many Catholics find it an important way to prepare for death or to lift feelings of guilt about unresolved personal issues. This sacrament can be administered only by a priest, who has unique legal protection to hear confidences in complete confidentiality. A nurse will want to facilitate patient privacy at such a moment.

Eucharist, a central sacrament for Roman Catholics, is also called "communion" or "the host." Observant Catholics receive the Eucharist weekly and on designated holy days. Some may wish to receive it as often as daily when they are sick. The Eucharist can be brought to the bedside if the patient cannot attend the worship service. When a person is "n.p.o" (not to eat or drink anything in preparation for surgery), the wafer can be touched to the lips. A nurse may call the chaplain's office to request the Eucharist for a patient or family member.

Special Concerns   *Devotional Materials.* Scapulars are small pictures of Mary or Jesus worn around the neck. When possible, they should not be removed during care. Rosary beads and pictures of Mary and the saints are important religious objects often placed at the bedside or brought from home. Families may wish to send them to surgery with a child, and care should be taken to prevent loss. Some devotional items have been passed down from one generation to another and cannot be replaced. Holy water, which comes from places such as the grotto at Lourdes, is highly regarded for its healing powers.

Family Planning. The Roman Catholic Church endorses the concept of "responsible parenthood" (Paul VI, 1968: no. 10) and a natural method of family planning that is based on the ovulation cycle. The church affirms that life begins at conception and therefore prohibits abortion and the use of abortive medication. Following the Catholic Church's teaching that married love is both unitive and procreative, contraceptive pills, medications, devices, and use of condoms are prohibited. Sterilization, including tubal ligation and vasectomy to prevent pregnancy, is also prohibited (Paul VI, 1968: no. 12, 13).

If, in a clinician's opinion, there are compelling medical reasons to consider pregnancy termination or the use of contraceptive devices, clinicians may suggest that the patient consult with her priest or the hospital's Catholic chaplain. The ethical principle of double effect may give the patient an opportunity to make a decision that is compatible with faith and conscience (Paul VI, 1968: no. 15).

Death. Because he is viewed as an intermediary between the believer and God, and one whose prayers have special merit, the priest is often requested at the time of death. Even when all sacramental care has been provided earlier, families may request that the priest be present.

Families may request an emergency baptism or Sacrament of the Sick prior to death (see above). The Catholic Church has a high regard for the preservation and dignity of life, including the sick, disabled, and unborn. The church does not obligate persons to pursue gravely burdensome or ineffective life-sustaining interventions. Analgesics may be used in sufficient amounts to relieve pain, even if life is thereby shortened, so long as death is not the intended effect.

Autopsy. There are no special concerns for postmortem care. Organ donation and autopsy are a matter of personal preference.

The Roman Catholic Church offers an extensive network of pastoral, social, and medical support services to assist individuals facing difficult issues associated with pregnancy.

References

Magida, A. J. (Ed.). (1996). Roman Catholicism. *How to be a perfect stranger.* Woodstock, NY: Jewish Lights Publishing.

Park Ridge Center for the Study of Health, Faith, and Ethics. (1996). *The Roman Catholic tradition: Religious beliefs and health care decisions.* Chicago, IL: Park Ridge Center.

Pope Paul VI. (1968). *Human vitae.* Rome, Italy: The Vatican.

Websites: *www.fas.harvard.edu/~pluralsm, www.christianity.net,* and *www. webcom.com/~nlnnet/xianres.html*

Santería

Introduction

This information is given as an introduction to a specific religious tradition and is meant to help providers understand similarities and variations among religious practices. Providers are cautioned not to overgeneralize or characterize all members of a religious group as alike. In fact, a person's spiritual and religious profile is unique and can be determined only when trust has been established and open-ended assessment questions have been asked.

The provider is encouraged to inquire about the family's spiritual needs near the end of an initial interview. Perhaps the topic can be introduced by saying: "We know that illness can be very stressful. Many families find their faith or spiritual beliefs a source of strength or comfort during a hospital stay. I'm wondering if your spirituality or religion is important to you?" If the patient or family says "yes," these questions follow naturally:[*]

"Do you follow a particular religious tradition or spiritual path?" If the answer is yes, "Would you like a visit from your own clergy or a hospital chaplain during your stay?" If the answer is yes, "Would you like to include that person in the conversation when it comes time to make an important treatment decision?"

Some other possible questions include the following:

- "Are there religious customs or spiritual practices that are important to you, but likely to be disrupted during this hospital stay or illness?"

- "Are there ways that we can help you maintain your spiritual strength or routine during this stay (for example, worship opportunities, medals, devotional materials, kosher meals, Sabbath candles, communion, baptism, prayer rug, and so forth)?"

- "How does your faith influence the way you think about this illness?"

When making an assessment, additional factors to consider include age, gender, ethnic group, developmental stage, family structure, faith community, life experiences, psychosocial history, and individual characteristics. Providers should consult the hospital chaplain for assistance with an assessment.

---

[*] These questions were adapted from L. Carpenito, *Nursing Diagnosis: Application to Clinical Practice* (7th ed.). New York: Lippincott Williams & Wilkins, 1997.

This information is about Santerían traditions and practices.

In Brief

- Santería is an African-based religious tradition that is practiced in Cuba and other Afro-Caribbean and Latin American countries. It is also practiced among some people in U.S. Latino communities.

- Santería comprises a mix of West African Yoruba, Catholicism, and French spiritism. This practice evolved in Cuba centuries ago among African slaves who were prohibited from practicing their native Yoruba in a predominantly Catholic setting. They hid the practice by identifying each "orisha" (spirit) with a Catholic saint. For example, Saint Peter is also "Ogun," the iron spirit.

- "Olodumare," or "Olofi," is the supreme God. Orishas are said to be intermediaries between Olofi and the human world.

- Many followers of Santería also practice other Christian religions.

- Patients and their families may have a blend of spiritual practices and may be hesitant to disclose this to providers or the Catholic chaplain.

Place of Worship

Followers worship in the house of a Santero or Santera.

Clergy

Santeros and Santeras are priests and priestesses who communicate with the orishas. The "Babalawo" is the high priest.

Worship Traditions

Divinations are performed by Santeros and Santeras reading sea shells, nuts, or rocks that are scattered on the floor or table. The orishas reveal their diagnoses and solutions to a person's problems through the patterns the objects create when thrown. People seek help from the Santeros and Santeras about issues such as health, interpersonal relationships, and finances.

Offerings are made to the orishas to give special thanks for their effective work. They are also an offering of good wishes for the saints. Glasses or bottles of rum or wine are popular offerings. Sacrifices are also made to the orishas for the same purposes. Sacrifices may include the slaughter and consumption of an animal (usually a chicken or pigeon). Each orisha is said to have its favorite offering.

Drum and dance festivals, known as "bembe," are also a form of offering to the orishas. During the drumming and dancing, participants are said to enter trances or a state of euphoria. During these trances the orishas are said to communicate with the Santero and other participants.

Religious Observance in the Hospital Setting

Worship   During a time of illness, the patient or family may wish to consult a Babalawo (high priest). The high priest will perform a special ceremony in the home to summon the highest powers to intervene on behalf of the patient. In rare situations a patient may request permission for a leave of absence for a few hours to participate in this ceremony.

Care of the Sick   *Pastoral Care.* Santeros may be sought for advice and spiritual guidance concerning issues of behavior, developmental problems, mental illness, and relationship and life issues. Typically, the patient or family will initiate this contact independently, in addition to seeing the hospital chaplain.

Pre-admission Preparation. A Santero may be asked to do a cleansing ceremony ("Ebbo") on the patient prior to admission for surgery. The Santero places a pigeon inside a bag and rubs the bag over the patient's body in an effort to spiritually cleanse the patient to remove "spirits of death." Requests for a Santero's treatment during a critical illness warrant careful consideration by hospital staff if the trust of the patient and family are to be maintained.

Treatment. Cleansing herbal baths, herbal teas, or objects of reverence may be used in conjunction with medical care to provide spiritual energy. They can be purchased at "botanicas," shops located in Latino communities.

Devotional Materials. Beaded necklaces or bracelets (that were given to a person during his or her spiritual initiation) are used to keep death away. Providers should avoid removal of such objects and consider sending them to surgery with the patient, if requested. Care should be taken to prevent loss.

Special Concerns   *Birth Defects.* Those who practice Santería may see genetic disorders and birth defects as a curse. They may desire spiritual investigation, spiritual cleansing, and herbal remedies in addition to medical interventions. The services of a Santero may well help such parents bond more effectively with their newborn and be more compliant with the medical regimen.

Organ Transplantation. Organ transplantation and donation may be viewed negatively; the entire body is considered to belong to the spirits. If organs are to be removed, special permission may be needed from the orishas before a decision can be made.

Death. At the time of death, a Babalawo or a Santero may be called to do a special cleansing ceremony prior to burial.

Autopsy and cremation are not permitted.

References

Lefever, H. (1996, September). When the saints go riding in: Santería in Cuba and the United States. Cuban religion. *The Journal for the Scientific Study of Religion, 35*(3), 318–330.

Murphy, J. (1988). *Santería: An African religion in America.* Boston, MA: Beacon Press.

Pasquali, E. (1994, December). Santería. *Journal of Holistic Nursing, 12*(4), 380–390.

Valdes, A. (1994, December 15). A faith emerges from the shadows. *Boston Globe,* p. 73.

Websites: *www.nando.net* and *www.orishanet.com/ochanet.html*

Rabbi Shapiro

IN THIS CASE STUDY ABOUT THE DEATH OF AN ORTHODOX Jewish patient, the staff recognized their sense of frustration with requests that seemed out of the ordinary and labor-intensive. Yet their knowledge of another's religious tradition and their respect for the spiritual needs of the patient and his family enabled them to fold spiritual sensitivity into their practice, resulting in superior care. Spiritual sensitivity is highly prized by the patient and family and is a source of professional satisfaction for the clinician. This case demonstrates that one does not need to share a cultural or religious tradition in order to honor a patient's preferences.

The emergency department phone rings, breaking the morning silence. An 82-year-old man with terminal brain cancer has been found unresponsive at home. Ten minutes later, he arrives in agonal breathing.

"Any family? Any DNR papers?" Lark, one of the registered nurses, asks of no one in particular as we move the patient to the cart. "His family is on the way," says one of the paramedics.

Lark assists in ventilating the patient while we strip off his clothes, revealing an Orthodox Jewish prayer garment. A collective sigh is audible.

Privately, we on the ED staff have discussed our frustrations with the restrictions of Orthodox Jewish religious beliefs regarding end-of-life issues. An Orthodox Jewish physician had explained the Orthodox perspective to us. He said some Orthodox Jews distinguish between not allowing a life-maintaining act to be performed and actually stopping an intervention that maintains life. Therefore, while some Orthodox Jews would allow discontinuation of manual ventilation (viewing this as passively allowing an illness to take its course), they would not necessarily permit a life-support machine to be turned off (viewing this as an act that deliberately ends life). In some Israeli hospitals, ventilators are equipped with timers, thus making the issue whether to reset the ventilator rather than whether to turn it off.

When the family arrives, we learn that the patient and family have never discussed an advance directive with their physician. I feel frustrated that clinicians never before approached the family about this issue at a less emotional time, given the patient's terminal condition. They say they want everything done for the patient, who's been identified as Rabbi Shapiro. I wonder if they understand what "everything" means.

It was a difficult intubation with multiple attempts. Dr. Dhawapun tells us, "Since Rabbi Shapiro is an Orthodox Jew, continue manually bagging him while I talk with the family. Given their probable religious beliefs, it might be impossible to take him off a ventilator once he's on."

His eyes are dilated, totally unresponsive. Blood pressure is sky-high; drips started. Foley catheter in. Labs drawn. X-ray taken. The usual measures are in place.

Minutes later, the patient's wife comes into the ED. "Isaac, can you hear me?" she asks calmly. The only response is the beeping from the tachycardiac rhythm monitor and the rhythmic whooshing of the ambu bag.

"I thought he'd be better by now," she says, turning to Dr. Dhawapun. "It's better to stop what you're doing."

"Sometimes it helps when you actually see the situation yourself," Dr. Dhawapun says softly.

I'm surprised. This isn't what I'd expected. I'm touched to be witnessing a moment of such raw human drama.

The patient's daughter and son-in-law are standing near the patient's wife. The daughter is sobbing. "Why don't we wait and see what happens over the next few days?" she says. "It's too soon to make a decision. We don't know what will happen."

My expectations were right after all, I think. *Status quo. All will continue.*

The family leaves with Dr. Dhawapun. When she returns, she informs us, "They want me to discuss the patient's condition with their rabbi."

Davis, the respiratory therapist, continues bagging, bagging, bagging. ED life goes on: Additional patients are admitted and discharged.

This story originally appeared as "Rest in Peace, Rabbi Shapiro" by Polly Gerber Zimmermann, in the *American Journal of Nursing,* April 1998, *98*(4), 64–65. © 1998 by Lippincott Williams & Wilkins. Reprinted with permission.

After a telephone conversation with the family's rabbi and further discussion with the family, Dr. Dhawapun tells us, "If the CT scan is positive for intracranial bleeding, the manual bagging can be stopped." Davis continues bagging, bagging, bagging. We are silent, caught up in the gravity of the situation as we work for a satisfactory resolution for all.

A half-hour later, Dr. Dhawapun gives the family the results. "I'm sorry, but the CT scan shows that there is massive bleeding throughout the brain," she explains.

The family agrees to stop the artificial ventilation. One by one, they say good-bye and leave, except for the son-in-law, who stays and takes out a prayer book.

After a total of 90 minutes of manually bagging the patient, Davis stops but remains in the room. The only sound is the heart monitor beeping. It always feels odd to do nothing in the presence of physical deterioration. As an ED nurse, I'm geared toward "fixing."

"Tell me when he is gone," the son-in-law says. "Of course," I say. I'm surprised by my own sadness. I find myself silently praying for the man and his family. Even when fully expected, it still is usually a shock to finally have the person "dead" instead of "dying."

I feel some nagging guilt for not leaving to care for the living, but the feeling quickly fades. I know I need to be here even though I only stand quietly with Davis at the patient's side.

The ET tube is still in place. "Can you take out that tube and save it in a bag for me? I don't think he's comfortable with it in," says the son-in-law.

Since Orthodox Jews usually request that anything containing body secretions be left undisturbed and buried with the patient, I'm startled by the son-in-law's request.

"Of course," I say.

"How long does he have?"

"It will be soon," Davis responds.

I inform the son-in-law of the impending end. "His heart rate is dropping, and his oxygen level is very low. He has some reflexive movements, but as you can see, his breathing isn't adequate."

In another 10 minutes, Rabbi Shapiro's pulse is down to three beats per minute. A minute later I tell his son-in-law, "His heart is no longer beating. He's gone."

This story originally appeared as "Rest in Peace, Rabbi Shapiro" by Polly Gerber Zimmermann, in the *American Journal of Nursing*, April 1998, *98*(4), 64–65. © 1998 by Lippincott Williams & Wilkins. Reprinted with permission.

The son-in-law asks to be alone for a few minutes. Davis and I leave the room. When I return, I detach and save the rest of the life support apparatus as requested. The *Chevra Kadisha*, holy group, will determine if it should be completely removed.

The family sits by the body until the Orthodox rabbi undertaker arrives.

"Ah, Rabbi Shapiro was a wonderful rabbi!" the undertaker shares with me. "So well respected in the community."

"It's always sad to lose a great man," I say. The undertaker leaves the room, forgetting the bloodied equipment. It has become extremely important to me that Rabbi Shapiro has what he needs when he's buried. I run down the hall and through the parking lot to give the equipment to the undertaker.

When I return to the ED nurses' station, the son-in-law comes over to thank us. I sincerely tell him how very sorry I am for his loss.

I've witnessed countless deaths in my nursing career. They are always sobering and affect me deeply. At different times, I feel sadness, relief, anger, or numbness. But this time I feel a rewarding, peaceful satisfaction.

It wasn't cost-effective or practical to perform extensive manual bagging when mechanical ventilation was available. But today, a Buddhist, a Catholic, and an Episcopalian worked together to help an Orthodox Jewish man have a dignified death that was consistent with his religious beliefs and those of his family.

We did a good thing.

References

Association of Orthodox Jewish Scientists, Raphael Society, Health Care Section. (1990). In F. Rosner (Ed.), *Medicine and Jewish law*. Northvale, NJ: J. Aronson.

Levin, F. (1987). *Halacha, medical science and technology: Perspectives on contemporary Halacha issues*. New York: Maznaim.

This story originally appeared as "Rest in Peace, Rabbi Shapiro" by Polly Gerber Zimmermann, in the *American Journal of Nursing*, April 1998, *98*(4), 64–65. © 1998 by Lippincott Williams & Wilkins. Reprinted with permission.

Part Three

Tools

Chapter 11

Utilizing Resources to Better Serve Multicultural Patients

Consultation on Cultural or Religious Issues

Cultural consultation may be available from a cadre of trained professionals within the hospital health care system.

Many members of the pastoral care, social work, psychiatric nursing, psychology, and psychiatry staff are trained to provide cultural consultation. Start by conferring with the pastoral care and/or mental health staff assigned to your unit or clinical program, who may be able to consult on cultural or religious issues.

Such consultants may offer knowledge of the culture gained through being a member of the culture and/or extensive experience working with individuals from specific cultural or religious traditions. They may be able to provide information about family structure and roles, health beliefs and practices, and immigration patterns and their impact on families. Consultants are skilled and trained in providing consultation to health care providers. The role of the consultant includes

- Providing factual information about the specific religious tradition and culture;

- Assisting the team in identifying and discussing with the patient and family any cultural traditions and health beliefs that could influence understanding of the diagnosis and care plan, as well as future compliance with recommendations for care at home;

- Assisting the team in incorporating knowledge of the patient and the family culture into both their assessment and treatment plan; and

- Assisting the team in dealing with misunderstandings or conflicts that may arise in the patient, family, and staff relationships due to cultural differences.

Interpreter Services

Many people feel more comfortable communicating in their native language. Interpreters can be very useful for communicating with patients and their families. Many times cultural consultation or cultural mediation is available from trained interpreters as part of their role as a member of the health care team. Interpreters are especially important for the following reasons:

- Although many immigrant families do have some command of the English language and use it in their daily lives, they may not understand the special vocabulary used in a hospital setting or for medical purposes. The information the patient conveys is often the basis for medical decisions that can have serious consequences for the health and well-being of the patient and his or her family. Mistakes or misunderstandings may jeopardize the patient's health and should be avoided.

- Illness can provoke fear and anxiety. This is especially true in emergency situations or when the matter to be discussed is of a delicate nature (complicated medical situations, venereal disease, family planning, abortion, or AIDS, for instance).

- Many people simply feel more comfortable communicating in their native language with the assistance of an interpreter.

- Using interpreters reduces legal risk. Their use may minimize potential liability because of inadequate informed consent, delay in receiving clinical intervention, and inappropriate treatment resulting from provider or family misunderstanding. Moreover, federal legislation prohibits discrimination against persons because of national origin or because of a primary language other than English. Effective interpreter services programs help to fulfill legal mandates against unlawful discrimination.

Finding the Appropriate Interpreter

Because monolingual providers are frequently unable to assess another person's language skills, they often assume that anyone who is more or less (or even fully) bilingual can act as an interpreter. On this basis, hospital employees, family members (other than the parents of a child), other patients, and in many cases children are called on to interpret. This can cause several problems. First, these individuals do not always understand the medical terminology being used and the importance of the information they are relaying. Second, they are not working under a code of ethical standards that would emphasize, for instance, the privacy and confidentiality of the information they are asked to convey or elicit. Third, family members, because of their emotional involvement, lack objectivity, and may be unable to interpret impartially without interjecting their own opinions and biases.

COSSHMO (1988) reported the following on the use of children as interpreters:

> The use of a child who interprets for his/her parents, whatever the setting, inverts the role that most cultures ascribe in the family hierarchy by putting the child in a temporarily superior position. Parents will hesitate to discuss intimate issues or conflicts in front of their children. A child will feel pressure to be accurate and clear in his/her interpretation and will become frustrated when unable to meet those expectations. The child may also feel ashamed of his/her parent. (p. 1)

A study conducted at Boston City Hospital compared encounters mediated by professional interpreters with encounters mediated by family members. When professional interpreters were used, fewer tests were ordered (as a result of a better understanding of the patient's complaint) and, on average, substantially less time was spent with the patient (Hardt, 1991).

When there is a language barrier, the individual used as an interpreter holds the keys to the communication process and wields considerable power. Cross-cultural interpretation requires special training and highly developed skills. Downing (1992) writes that some of these skills include

> a broad knowledge of both languages and the cultures in which they are spoken; an ability to grasp readily and completely what others say in either language; an ability to speak in either language so as to be readily understood; a good memory for what is heard; the ability to find semantically and culturally equivalent means of expression in each language, even when there are no equivalent words; a knowledge of specialized vocabulary in areas such as medicine and the law and of the concepts and systems behind them, as well as of variant social and dialectical forms of expression that may be used by clients; and the ability to maintain consistent accuracy in rendering the interpretation. (p. 7)

The role of the interpreter is to make possible optimal communication between provider and patient when there is a language and/or cultural barrier. A trained professional interpreter, in addition to having the necessary skills for the job, has a clear understanding of his or her role, knows the importance of remaining in that role, and follows a code of ethics.

The Massachusetts Medical Interpreters Association's Code of Ethics for interpreters dictates

> that all assignment related information is private and confidential; that the interpreter must interpret impartially, accurately, and completely the spirit and content of each speaker; that the interpreter shall act as a cultural broker and communicate the patient's cultural and social context as it relates to medical needs, and/or may affect the type of therapy or treatment; that the interpreter shall not accept assignments that are beyond his or her language or subject competency, or where there is a potential conflict of interest; and that the interpreter shall strive to further professional skills and knowledge.

Medical Interpretation as a Profession

Although the court system has had interpreter training and certification programs in place for some time, today only a handful of programs in the United States train medical interpreters, and no states require any type of professional regulation or certification. This is slowly changing across the country as health care facilities begin to realize the need and benefits of having trained medical interpreters.

In Massachusetts, for example, interpreters from many hospitals have organized into the Massachusetts Medical Interpreters Association (MMIA). The association has developed the first Medical Interpreting Standards of Practice. These standards, which have been recognized as a model document by many states, provide a defining baseline of expectations for consumers and practitioners and establish criteria for certification and/or entry into the profession, ensuring quality and consistency of performance. Copies of the Standards of Practice can be ordered from the MMIA. The association is currently working to develop a certification process for medical interpreters (MMIA, 1998).

In addition to making interpreters available in the languages most commonly spoken by the patient population served, some of the goals of any interpreter services program, according to the MMIA, should be

> to provide ongoing training to staff in cross-cultural issues and how to work effectively with interpreters; to provide ongoing training to interpreters to further their professional skills and knowledge; and to monitor the interpreting needs of the patient population served and adapt the program accordingly.

Using Interpreters Effectively

Having an interpreter present adds a third person to the provider-patient dyad. A successful interpreter-mediated interview is only possible when there is a good balance of power, when provider, interpreter, and patient work as partners.

For the interpreter, this means recognizing and respecting the provider's expertise and allowing him or her to direct the interview; not expressing personal beliefs or opinions unless the interpreter's input is necessary to offer cultural insights; never giving medical advice on his or her own; assuring the patient that all the information will remain confidential; and respecting the patient's right to make his or her own decisions.

For the provider, this means including the interpreter as a member of the health care team and empowering the interpreter in his or her field of expertise, communication—that is, allowing him or her to mediate the flow of the conversation, to input relevant information as a "cultural broker," to use the most effective mode of interpretation, and to suggest the best seating arrangement of parties.

Tips for Working with Non-English-Speaking Patients

The following tips will help providers working with non-English-speaking patients:

- Use an interpreter when the limited English proficiency of the patient and/or parent(s) or your own limited ability to speak their language can result in a compromise of the patient's right to access appropriate health care services.

- Avoid using children, family members, hospital employees (unless they have been recruited, trained, and referred by hospital interpreter services), or other patients just because they are bilingual.

- Request a trained interpreter from within the hospital's interpreter program. Ideally, the facility's program should provide in-house coverage for languages in high demand, have a staff person on call twenty-four hours a day, and have access to a pool of freelance interpreters in the languages most commonly spoken in the area.

- Whenever possible meet briefly with the interpreter to offer some background information and discuss the goals and expectations for the interview prior to meeting with the patient.

- Directly address the patient when in conversation. Talk through the interpreter, not *to* the interpreter.

00:00:2200:00:21

- Remember that the interpreter, as a communications facilitator, is only relaying messages of others. A good interpreter will convey, unedited and unpolished, the patient's jargon, language level, anecdotal information, or even failure to respond directly to a question. Interpreters should translate everything that is said in both directions.

- Take advantage of the interpreter's knowledge of the culture. The patient and family's cultural beliefs and traditions may be an important component in the illness and its treatment. Medical treatment, child care and discipline, and nutrition habits can be culture-dependent.

- Providers who work frequently with a specific linguistic and cultural group would benefit from education about the group's historical and sociopolitical background and about diseases and illnesses of high incidence among its members.

Strategies for Conversations with the Patient and Family

- Speak in short sentences, emphasizing one point or asking one question at a time.

- Break lengthy explanations into shorter ideas and ask the interpreter to explain them one at a time.

- Avoid medical or technical jargon that is not easily understood by the patient.

Informed Consent

It is the provider's role, not the interpreter's, to fully explain any procedure for which consent is required. Ask the interpreter to translate all components of the consent form, rather than simply asking for the signature.

References

COSSHMO. (1988, January). Across cultures: Tips for health care providers. *National Coalitions of Hispanic Health and Human Services, 2*(4).

Downing, B.T. (1992). *Professional interpretation: Insuring access for refugee and immigrant patients.* Minneapolis, MN: Department of Linguistics, University of Minnesota.

Hardt, E. (1991). *The bilingual medical interview.* Boston, MA: Boston City Hospital and the Boston Area Health Education Center.

Massachusetts Medical Interpreters Association, New England Medical Center, 750 Washington Street, NEMC Box 271, Boston, MA 02111–1845; 617-636-5479.

Pastoral Care

Hospital chaplains often provide religious consultation or mediation. The chaplain can clarify spiritual concerns in the health care setting and assist both providers and family members in seeking a plan of care that is medically appropriate and sensitive to religious issues.

Other Members of the Health Care Team

Ancillary staff members may share their knowledge of a culture and its health beliefs that they have gained through being a member of that culture or through training. This level of consultation is considered a part of their professional roles.

External Consultants

Experts outside of the health care organization may provide in-service education regarding specific cultures or may be asked to comment from their knowledge base in a range of case-based training situations.

For more information about how to coordinate with external organizations, refer to the next chapter. Local and national human service agencies may be able to provide information about particular cultures or religious traditions or be able to provide direct assistance to patients and families who are looking for help with emergency food or shelter, English as a Second Language (ESL) classes, citizenship, legalization or amnesty counseling, and employment. Social workers within the health care institution should maintain a list of agencies to which they can refer patients and families, such as local chapters of the American Red Cross, Catholic Charities, United Way, or international language schools. Some possible resource agencies are listed in the References and Other Resources section at the end of this book.

Templates to collect information about cultural or religious traditions that may be relevant in the health care setting are provided on the following pages.

Template for Collecting Cultural Information

Introduction

This information is given as an introduction to a specific culture and is meant to help providers understand similarities and variations in cultural practices. Providers are cautioned not to overgeneralize or characterize all members of a cultural or ethnic group as alike. Factors to be considered in assessing a person's cultural identity and his or her actions or beliefs include individual characteristics, socioeconomic status, race, education, religion, age, gender, the stages, conditions, and adjustment to the migration experience, and whether the family came from a rural or urban area.

This sheet is about _____ traditions and practices.

Country of Origin and Geographic Location

Language

Migration Patterns

Are there political or economic conditions that might affect the patient's mental or physical health?

Spiritual Traditions

How are spiritual practices affected in the health care setting?

Family

Include information on the immigrant group's marriage patterns, gender roles, family and kinship structure, and intergenerational issues.

Diet and Nutrition

Include any foods that are not eaten, as well as those preferred in times of illness and other foods used to promote health and well-being.

Attitudes and General Beliefs
About Illness and Death

Implications for Providers

Cultural Courtesies

Include any relevant information for the health care setting.

Communication Patterns and Value Orientation

Include method of greeting, and particular issues concerning gestures, personal space, or body language.

Traditional Medical Practices

Describe known practices that may be incorporated into a plan of care.

Other Issues Relevant to Hospitalization

Discuss issues such as autopsy, organ transplantation, blood loss and donation, or views concerning death.

References

Be sure to ask other members of the cultural tradition to help write the information and to serve as proofreaders.

Template for Collecting Information About Religious Traditions

Introduction

This information is given as an introduction to a specific religious tradition and is meant to help providers understand similarities and variations among religious practices. Providers are cautioned not to overgeneralize or characterize all members of a religious group as alike. In fact, a person's spiritual and religious profile is unique and can be determined only when trust has been established and open-ended assessment questions have been asked.

The provider is encouraged to inquire about the family's spiritual needs near the end of an initial interview. Perhaps the topic can be introduced by saying: "We know that illness can be very stressful. Many families find their faith or spiritual beliefs a source of strength or comfort during a hospital stay. I'm wondering if your spirituality or religion is important to you?" If the patient or family says "yes," these questions follow naturally:*

"Do you follow a particular religious tradition or spiritual path?" If the answer is yes, "Would you like a visit from your own clergy or a hospital chaplain during your stay?" If the answer is yes, "Would you like to include that person in the conversation when it comes time to make an important treatment decision?"

Some other possible questions include the following:

- "Are there religious customs or spiritual practices that are important to you, but likely to be disrupted during this hospital stay or illness?"

- "Are there ways that we can help you maintain your spiritual strength or routine during this stay (for example, worship opportunities, medals, devotional materials, kosher meals, Sabbath candles, communion, baptism, prayer rug, and so forth)?"

- "How does your faith influence the way you think about this illness?"

When making an assessment, additional factors to consider include age, gender, ethnic group, developmental stage, family structure, faith community, life experiences, psychosocial history, and individual characteristics. Providers should consult the hospital chaplain for assistance with an assessment.

---

* These questions were adapted from L. Carpenito, *Nursing Diagnosis: Application to Clinical Practice* (7th ed.). New York: Lippincott Williams & Wilkins, 1997.

The following information sheet is about _____ practices and traditions.

In Brief

Provide the history, underlying principles, and definitions of terms in the religious practice.

Place of Worship

Do members join together for worship in a temple, a church, a meeting house?

Clergy

What are members of the clergy called and what is their function?

Holy Days

What are the days with religious significance, and do they affect health care?

Religious Observance in the Hospital Setting

Worship

How is religion practiced in the health care setting?

Dietary Needs

Are there dietary requirements or preferences, always or on certain days, and how do these affect health care?

Care of the Sick

Describe the role of pastoral care in the health care facility and how the provider can communicate with a religious leader.

Describe the role of prayer and how the provider can assist in the health care setting.

Discuss how different treatment options may be seen by the patient or his or her family.

Special Concerns

Include religious policies regarding autopsy, organ donation and transplantation, abortion, birth, blood transfusions and blood products, death, postmortem care, cremation or burial rituals, and any special funeral preparations required.

References

Be sure to use lay members and clergy from the specific group, as well as local churches or religious organizations, as consultants and to proofread your work.

Chapter 12

Meeting Joint Commission Standards Related to Culture and Religion

Understanding the unique influence of culture and religion for an individual and his or her family is an essential component of good patient care. It can impact a patient's perception of the health care experience, as well as affect compliance and treatment outcomes.

Essential elements of a culturally competent health care organization include standards, policies and procedures that support patient preferences, trained and sensitive staff, comprehensive interpreter services, multicultural resources, multilingual teaching materials, availability of a chaplain, an environment of understanding and respect, and thorough medical record documentation.

The Joint Commission on Accreditation of Healthcare Organizations (JCAHO) emphasizes the importance of honoring patients' cultural and religious preferences in several standards published in *Assessment of Patients, Care of Patients, Patient and Family Education,* and *Patient Rights.* The commission recognizes that culture and religion often play a pivotal role in patient assessment, treatment, education, and participation in care. The intent of these standards is to ensure that the broad needs of patients are considered and that patients receive individualized, appropriate care.

Although culture and religion are explicitly referred to in only a few of the JCAHO standards, many others contain cultural and religious implications. During an accreditation survey, an organization's compliance with the standards and their intent is evaluated, and the organization must demonstrate that it is meeting the psychosocial, emotional, and spiritual needs of its patients. Overall compliance must be demonstrated by verbal information, surveyor observation, and documentation (Joint Commission, 1998).

Proper documentation of cultural and religious care facilitates meaningful team communication and can indicate an institution's quality practice and how a JCAHO standard is being met. When documenting information about culture and religion, all relevant facts should be captured. This includes information that may affect patient understanding, treatment, and compliance. Clinicians should note significant comments, observed behaviors of the patient and family, staff interventions, physician notifications, interpreters involved, and any referrals made to religious support persons and community agencies (Summer, 1998). Clinicians should use nonjudgmental terms and avoid vague and subjective wording that may lead to misinterpretation. Using direct quotations helps keep entries objective. Many types of documentation forms can be used to capture this information, but more important than the form is the content.

Thorough documentation can also assist with meeting standards for other regulatory agencies, such as Medicaid. The content of entries, behavioral terms used, and integration within the total context of care all contribute to effective documentation (Cornett, 1993).

Some examples of Boston Children's Hospital's policies, procedures, guidelines, and standards related to culture and religion are contained in the Appendix. These are only an example of one approach an organization can undertake to set expectations for staff regarding cultural and religious care. The documents can also support a hospital's compliance with JCAHO standards that refer to culture and religion. Included in the Appendix are the following policy and standards documents:

Standard for Nursing Practice: Culture and Care

Emergency Baptism Procedures

Ethics Committee Consultation

Ethics of Redirecting Goals of Care

Religious Objections to Blood Transfusions

Organ and Tissue Donation

Patient and Family Education

The following pages outline JCAHO standards related to culture and religion. They are organized by topic. Case examples and sample medical record documentation are also given. The examples cited represent nine actual and six composite cases. Details have been altered to protect patient and staff confidentiality.

Assessment of Patients

Standard PE.1: "Each patient's physical, psychological, and social status are assessed" (Joint Commission, 1998, p. 61).

Relationship to Culture and Religion

Culture and religion may play an important role in a patient's response to illness and treatment. The impact of these influences must be assessed when a patient is admitted to the hospital or visits an outpatient setting (Joint Commission, 1998, p. 61). For more information, see the section on Strategies for Providers in the Introduction, page xxiv.

Case Example

A three-day-old infant girl was admitted to the emergency department with a high fever. As the medical team prepared to draw blood, perform a spinal tap, and insert an intravenous line, the parents became markedly apprehensive and anxious. The nurse questioned the parents about their fears. As recent immigrants to this country from India, they were unfamiliar with the health care system in the United States and said that they had seen many infants die in their country before they reached their first birthday. The nurse explained that a fever does not necessarily mean a life-threatening illness. She described the rationale for each one of the tests and interventions and informed the family that early treatment with antibiotics decreases the risk for serious illnesses, such as bacteremia and meningitis. The nurse then communicated information about her interaction to the physician, who reinforced the explanations when he spoke with the family. The parents' fears were greatly alleviated.

Comments

Through careful questioning, the nurse was able to determine that the parent's anxiety was greater than usual for an emergency department visit and related to their cultural background. She provided the appropriate education and support and communicated her assessment to other team members.

Sample Medical Record Documentation

"Parents emigrated from India two years ago and are fluent in English. Both parents have graduate degrees and are not in need of financial assistance. Mother and father expressed fears that their child might die. Mother stated, 'In India, there is a high infant mortality rate, and many children die in the first year of life. Many illnesses start with a fever.' Family educated about spinal taps, blood cultures, and antibiotic therapy. Parents state they understand the need for tests and therapy and are less anxious."

Standard PF.1.1: "The assessment considers cultural and religious practices, emotional barriers, desire and motivation to learn, physical and cognitive limitations, language barriers, and the financial implications of care choices" (Joint Commission, 1998, p. 108).

Relationship to Culture and Religion

In a patient assessment, providers must identify cultural and religious practices that may impact hospitalization, treatment, and compliance. This cultural assessment data is then used for planning care. Beliefs, values, and practices can be structured into one of three categories: those that are beneficial to the treatment plan and should be continued, those that are neither harmful or helpful but can be incorporated into the plan, and those that are injurious and should be redirected (Narayan, 1997, p. 669).

Case Example

The infant child of Orthodox Jewish parents was being admitted to the hospital for treatment of an infection. The occupancy was near full, and the patient was assigned to a four-bed room by the patient placement coordinator. During the initial patient assessment, the nurse learned that the parents were observant Orthodox Jews. Further inquiry about their needs revealed that the mother was breast-feeding and planned to stay at the bedside overnight. In addition, the father had a daily practice of prayer in the morning, afternoon, and evening. The nurse was knowledgeable about Orthodox Jewish traditions and understood that a married woman could not sleep in the same room with an adult male who was not her husband. (See Chapter 10 for more information on Judaism.) She was also aware that privacy is important during prayer time. She spoke with the placement coordinator and some bed changes were made. The child was placed in a two-bed room in the space farthest from the door where the other sleep-in parent was a woman. A small refrigerator was obtained for Kosher foods, and directions were given to assist the family in using stairs, rather than elevators to maintain their Sabbath observance, when no electricity can be used.

Comments

The initial bed placement plan would have interfered with the spiritual needs of this family. The nurse was knowledgeable about Orthodox Jewish traditions and properly assessed the family's needs and concerns. She was able to intervene and work toward a more suitable arrangement.

Sample Medical Record Documentation

"Parents of child state, 'We are observant Orthodox Jews.' Mother requested single room, if possible, or a two-bed room. Mother cannot sleep in a room where an adult male is sleeping. Patient placed in two-bed room with a female parent near the window where curtain can be drawn. Small refrigerator obtained for patient's Kosher meals. Parents informed of availability of Jewish chaplain. Parent given bell to ring in lieu of call light on the Sabbath."

Patient and Family Education

Standard PF. 1.3: "Patients are educated about the safe and effective use of medication according to the law and their needs" (Joint Commission, 1998, p. 108).

Relationship to Culture and Religion

Providers must understand a patient's religious and cultural beliefs with regard to medications so this understanding can be taken into consideration when teaching is done. Misunderstandings about medications may affect a patient's compliance with the prescribed regimen.

Case Example

A twelve-year-old Haitian child was admitted to the mental health unit with a diagnosis of psychosis. When asked what they believed caused the illness, the family members told the provider that a spell had been cast on their child. As the provider discussed treatment, which included psychotropic medication, the family was very wary. They wanted to have the child exorcised by a Catholic priest. With the help of a Haitian physician from the community, the team educated the parents about the benefits of antipsychotic medications and urged them to see what the effect would be.

They also discussed side effects and ways to minimize them. In addition, the team arranged for a priest to come to the patient's hospital room and perform an exorcism. Within a few weeks, the child's condition had improved.

Comments

Mental illness is not well accepted by many Haitians and is believed to have supernatural causes (Colin & Paperwala, 1996). In this situation, with proper education and sensitivity toward their cultural beliefs, team members helped the family understand the importance of antipsychotic medication. In addition, the team was able to complement traditional Western treatment with the family's treatment of choice.

Sample Medical Record Documentation

"Twelve-year-old Haitian boy admitted to mental health unit. Parents stated, 'A spell has been cast on our child,' and initially refused medication for the child. Requested that a priest be allowed to come to the hospital to perform an exorcism. Dr. C., the attending physician, and Dr. L., from the community, spoke at length to the family about treatment and the need for antipsychotic medication. Family agreed to medical treatment after arrangements for exorcism made."

Standard PF.1.5: "Patients are educated about potential drug-food interactions and provided counseling on nutrition and modified diets" (Joint Commission, 1998, p. 108).

Relationship to Culture and Religion

Food is an integral part of culture, and ethnic factors strongly influence eating patterns and food preparation methods (Samolsky et al., 1990). Providers must be knowledgeable about a patient's food preferences related to culture in order to make appropriate nutritional recommendations.

Case Example

A seventeen-year-old girl was referred to a nutritionist for counseling by her primary care provider. Nine months earlier, she had moved from Puerto Rico to Massachusetts and gained 35 pounds in those months. She also reported that she was less active because of colder weather. Her provider had recommended that she try eating fish, salads, and plain baked potatoes, but the girl was unable to follow this plan.

After asking for a twenty-four-hour recall of foods eaten, the nutritionist learned that this adolescent was skipping breakfasts and lunches. She drank several cups of soda and juice during the day. After school, she usually was hungry and ate a large meal that her mother prepared. This meal consisted of one to two cups of rice, half a cup of beans, fried chicken wings, and fried plantains. Later in the evening, around 7 p.m., the girl joined her family for dinner, which included more rice and beans.

The nutritionist further questioned the patient about choices available at her school for lunch. There were many "fast food" items, but also turkey, ham, cheese, and tuna salad sandwiches. The nutritionist wanted to know how foods were prepared at home, but the girl did not know exactly what her mother added to various dishes. At this point, the nutritionist asked for permission to call the girl's mother and learned that she added large amounts of oil to most dishes.

The Puerto Rican diet consists mainly of rice, beans, starchy tubers, fried plantains, and sausage (Lang, 1992). The nutritionist was aware of this and the hidden fats in traditional foods. Her recommendations included eating breakfast, such as cereal with a banana and milk or one egg with toast and hot cocoa; selecting a sandwich for lunch; decreasing juice and soda intake and increasing water intake; delaying the 3 p.m. meal until 5 p.m. and eating one meal instead of two. She gave the mother some traditional recipes that called for less oil and more vegetables. With these modest changes, the girl began to lose weight gradually over the next few weeks.

Comments

The initial recommendations made by the primary care provider were met with resistance and noncompliance. A thorough assessment by the nutritionist identified the patient's dietary habits, and she made recommendations that helped the teen modify, but not completely change these habits. Working with her patient's cultural food preferences, this nutritionist was able to make individualized dietary suggestions that were appropriate for this situation.

Sample Medical Record Documentation

"Seventeen-year-old Puerto Rican girl referred for nutritional counseling due to thirty-five-pound weight gain in nine months. Current diet consists of no breakfast or lunch, large meal of rice, beans, fried chicken, and fried plantains after school, and dinner of rice and beans. Recommendations include not skipping meals, eating an egg or cereal for breakfast, selecting a healthy meal for lunch, and eating one meal at 5 p.m. Suggested decreasing oil in cooking and adding some frozen vegetables. Patient stated, 'I think I can do this.' Will monitor progress every two weeks."

Standard PF. 1.7: "Patients are informed about access to additional resources in the community" (Joint Commission, 1998, p. 108).

Relationship to Culture and Religion

Providers need to be aware of ethnic community resources. Community resources dedicated to specific patient populations can better meet their needs. (See Chapter 11.)

Case Example

A young woman from El Salvador became pregnant shortly after immigrating to the United States. A year later she became pregnant again, this time with twins. The twins were born prematurely, and one had complex medical needs. After a prolonged hospital stay, the infant was ready for discharge. The hospital social worker referred the mother to a social service agency that specialized in working with Spanish-speaking persons. The social worker obtained a case manager to help the mother cope with her social and financial needs, which included homelessness, unemployment, lack of financial resources, and lack of support systems. The case worker arranged for numerous services, including housing at a Spanish-speaking shelter, family therapy with a Spanish-speaking social worker, and Spanish-speaking primary care providers for her children.

Comments

During the hospital stay of the infant, the social worker identified the numerous social needs of this mother. The social worker was very knowledgeable about agencies in the community and was able to make a referral to one agency that could address all of the issues this mother had.

Sample Medical Record Documentation

"Spanish-speaking mother from El Salvador with numerous social needs, including homelessness, unemployment, lack of financial resources, and lack of support systems. Referred to La Agencia. Case manager arranging housing, primary care, and family therapy before discharge of infant son from NICU."

Standard PF. 1.9: *"The hospital makes clear to patients and families what their responsibilities are regarding the patient's ongoing health needs and gives them the knowledge and skills they need to carry out their responsibilities"* (Joint Commission, 1998, p. 109).

Relationship to Culture and Religion

Family roles and relationships vary from culture to culture. Providers must understand a family's roles, relationships, and support systems in planning education related to health needs. The Joint Commission (1998) emphasizes individualized strategies to help patients and families understand the importance of providing accurate information, asking questions, and carrying out instructions.

Case Example

An eight-year-old girl with an imperforate anus had a colostomy at birth. She was admitted to the hospital for a closure of her colostomy and an ileoanal pull through to create an anus. Accompanied by her father, she had traveled from United Arab Emirates for this surgery. Both the patient and her father were Muslim and spoke Arabic. Part of the post-operative care for this surgery involves dilating the rectum with a metal dilator twice each day for two months to ensure patency and to prevent obstruction. Caregivers are taught this procedure before discharge. For teaching sessions, an interpreter was used, but the father resisted and refused to perform the procedure. Days passed, and the father continued to refuse to carry out the rectal dilatations. Through the interpreter, the nurses explained the rationale over and over again. This strategy did little to change the father's behavior.

The interpreter, who was familiar with Muslim culture and traditions, realized that cultural issues were most likely having an impact on this situation. (See Chapter 10 for more information on the Muslim religion.) All the staff interacting with the father, including the interpreter, were women. In some cultures interactions between genders are proscribed. This Muslim father may have been unaccustomed to taking direction from a woman and probably felt uncomfortable with this. This presented a challenge for the staff and family.

In Muslim culture women assume the care-giving functions in the family; this role was probably new for the father. Modesty and privacy are highly respected, which could make performing the rectal dilatations exceptionally uncomfortable for the father, as well as for the daughter. The nurses and interpreter requested that the male surgeon talk to the father with a male Muslim physician translating. Together they explained the rationale for the procedure and consequences of not doing it. After a lengthy discussion, the father agreed and said he would instruct the mother in the dilatation procedure upon their return home. Within two weeks the patient was ready for discharge, and the staff felt comfortable that she would receive proper care.

Comments

In this very complex case, culture played an important role. Cultural mores of this family impacted the health care needs of the child. However, by accommodating the father's need to balance the customs of his religious tradition with the needs of his child, the important information was successfully communicated.

Sample Medical Record Documentation

"Practicing Muslim father and daughter, Arabic speaking with minimal English. Father instructed in post-op care, including rectal dilatations. Female Arabic interpreter used. Father refused to participate in several teaching sessions where procedure was demonstrated and rationale explained. Father declined to give reasons for his refusal. Attending surgeon, Dr. John X., accompanied by Dr. Al Y., a Muslim physician who translated, spoke at length to the father about the need for this procedure and potential negative outcomes if not followed. Father successfully performed procedure. Plan: have father dilate again tomorrow; have Dr. X communicate all critical information."

Standard PF.2: "Patient education is interactive" (Joint Commission, 1998, p. 110).

Relationship to Culture and Religion

A patient's culture may affect his or her understanding of health care information. During the education process, a provider needs to continuously elicit feedback to ensure that the patient receives the message.

Case Example

A one-year-old Japanese boy was admitted for a surgical repair involving his gastrointestinal tract. Diarrhea is a common post-operative complication, and care involves vigilant protection of the skin on the buttocks to prevent breakdown. Applications of therapeutic cream and powder were prescribed on a regular schedule. To preserve skin integrity, no soap or diaper wipes were allowed, and only ointment stained with stool was to be gently removed with each diaper change. Every twenty-four hours, the buttocks were soaked, and cream and powder were reapplied.

The mother, who spoke English, listened and nodded as the nurses explained the care and its rationale. However, after each diaper change, she was found washing her son's bottom in a basin. The nurse questioned her reasons for doing this, and the mother answered, "It's dirty." Further explanations by the nursing staff did not seem to change the mother's behavior. After consulting a resource on Japanese culture, the nurse learned that cleanliness is highly valued by the Japanese and believed to be linked to purification of the body and restoration of health (Shiba & Oka, 1996). She also learned that many Japanese are not comfortable with direct eye contact, commonly used by North American nurses during teaching sessions. She approached the mother without making direct eye contact and asked, "What worries you about this treatment?" The mother revealed that she feared her son would not recover if he were not kept clean. The nurse carefully explained the risk of skin breakdown and potential for infection, and asked for feedback to check the mother's understanding. The skin care plan was modified, and the mother was taught to soak her child's buttocks in a special solution every twelve hours. Then the cream and powder were reapplied. The mother complied with this regimen, and her son recovered without any skin breakdown.

Comments

Truly interactive patient education incorporates the patient's and family's health beliefs and concerns. Patient educators must ensure understanding by asking the patient or family to verbally repeat and demonstrate what they have learned (Joint Commission, 1998). In this case, once misunderstandings were clarified and the mother's concerns addressed, the plan of care was carried out.

Sample Medical Record Documentation

"Patient's mother of Japanese origin. Mother stated her concern that the cream preparation was 'dirty' and that she feared this may affect her son's recovery. Rationale for skin care regimen carefully explained, including risk for skin breakdown and infection. Mother taught to give Aveeno® soaks every twelve hours."

Standard PF.4: "The hospital identifies and provides the educational resources required to achieve its educational objectives" (Joint Commission, 1998, p. 111).

Relationship to Culture and Religion

A hospital that serves patients of different cultures must make educational materials available in appropriate languages. Interpreters must be available to work with providers, patients, and families during health care education sessions.

Case Example

An eleven-year-old Latino boy was receiving treatment for asthma. Although he was fluent in English, his mother spoke only a few words of this language. Her primary language was Spanish. When preparing for a teaching session regarding environmental triggers and asthma medications, the nurse arranged for a Spanish-speaking interpreter to be present. Teaching materials in both English and Spanish were given to both the mother and son.

Comments

Patient teaching should be provided in the primary language of the learner. In this situation, teaching was needed in both English and Spanish to meet the patient's and the family's needs. Written materials in the appropriate language offer reinforcement.

Sample Medical Record Documentation

"Asthma teaching regarding environmental triggers and medications done with patient and his mother. Spanish interpreter translated information for the mother. Mother able to state the triggers that affect her son and demonstrate proper use of nebulizer. Patient needs additional teaching about when to use nebulizer. Breathe Easier Spanish packet reviewed with mother. English version reviewed with patient."

Care of Patients

Standard TX.4.6: "The nutrition care service meets patients' needs for special diets and accommodates altered diet schedules" (Joint Commission, 1998, p. 89).

Relationship to Culture and Religion

Food preferences are typically culturally based. Health care institutions must be able to provide for the diverse nutritional needs of the populations they serve.

Case Example

An in-patient dietitian was consulted by nursing to see a four-year-old patient from India who had undergone cardiac surgery. The nurses noted that the patient was eating poorly, taking in only chocolates and water. The parents stated that their daughter normally consumed three meals a day plus snacks of traditional Indian food, including rice with lentils, curds, and a tortilla type of flat bread. The parents indicated difficulty in choosing foods from the hospital menu based on their daughter's lack of familiarity with the American diet.

The dietician worked with the family to develop a multifaceted plan. First, the parents and patient were informed of available foods similar to their usual diet, such as rice, beans, pita bread, and salad. Food choices were expanded to include the cafeteria menu for additional variety. Next, a volunteer of Indian descent who worked with the patient room service meal program visited with the patient and offered some home-cooked Indian food. Last, the dietitian provided education on ways to increase the caloric/nutritional density of the diet and initiated a high-calorie nourishing chocolate supplement. Two frappes daily provided approximately 85 percent of the child's caloric requirements. Within a week, the child's appetite improved, and she was receiving sufficient caloric and protein requirements for her age and size.

Comments

Adequate nutrition is an essential component of recovery and healing. In this situation, the patient was not receiving proper amounts of protein, carbohydrates, and calories because of her family's lack of familiarity with American foods. With proper management and planning, the nutrition service was able to provide ethnically appropriate foods and ensure adequate nutrition.

Sample Medical Record Documentation

"Four-year-old girl from India traveled to Children's with parents for cardiac surgery. Patient is now four days post-op and is noted by nurses to have poor appetite. Weight in fifth percentile for age. Parents report that their child is unfamiliar with the selections on the food service menu and does not like them. Patient prefers traditional Indian foods, such as rice, lentils, and pita bread. Patient menus planned to include these foods. Parents informed of cafeteria selections with ethnic appeal. Indian volunteer called and visited with patient. Volunteer to bring in home-cooked Indian meals. High-calorie chocolate frappes to be delivered twice a day. Parents agree with plan. Will monitor patient daily."

Standard TX.5.2.2: "*Discussions with the patient and family about the need for, risk of, and alternatives to blood transfusions when blood or blood components may be needed are considered*" (Joint Commission, 1998, p. 91).

Standard RI.1.2: "*Patients are involved in all aspects of their care*" (Joint Commission, 1998, p. 49).

Relationship to Culture and Religion

Care of patients requires a respect for religious and cultural beliefs. Patients' cultural and religious beliefs may affect how they participate in their care. Institutions and providers need to facilitate patients' and families' expression of their cultural and religious practices, so long as there is no harm to the patient or others (Joint Commission, 1998).

Case Example

An eight-year-old girl was to be admitted for a tonsillectomy and adenoidectomy (T & A). During her pre-operative assessment, the nurse asked if family members followed a particular religion or spiritual path. The father replied that they were practicing Jehovah's Witnesses. (See Chapter 10 for more information about Jehovah's Witness religious traditions.) Aware that followers of this religion may refuse blood transfusions and, although it is a rare complication of a T & A, a significant blood loss could occur, the nurse notified the anesthesiologist and together they engaged the parents in a discussion about their preferences regarding blood transfusions. The parents requested that their daughter not receive whole blood, red blood cells, or plasma but agreed to albumin, colloids, and crystalloids for volume expansion. A plan was made to use these alternative agents, if needed, and the consent form was amended to reflect this. The parents were informed that every effort would be made to avoid blood administration; however, in the event of a life-threatening situation, staff would seek a court order to authorize a blood transfusion. The parents agreed to the surgery, and the services of a chaplain were offered for spiritual support.

Comments

The parents were involved in deciding on acceptable blood alternatives. The hospital accommodated their request so long as there was no danger to the child. In the case of a competent adult patient, the patient's wishes would be honored, even in the event of an emergency.

Sample Medical Record Documentation

"Family members are practicing Jehovah's Witnesses. Parents request that patient not receive any blood transfusions. Alternatives discussed and agreed to—albumin, colloids, and crystalloids. Surgical consent form amended to reflect this. Parents informed that although every effort will be made to avoid a transfusion, in the event of a life-threatening emergency, a court order authorizing a blood transfusion would be obtained. Parents consented to the surgery and stated they understood the risks and benefits. Referral made to chaplain for spiritual support in the event of a transfusion."

Standard TX.5.2: "Before obtaining informed consent, the risks, benefits, and potential complications associated with procedures are discussed with the patient and family" (Joint Commission, 1998, p. 91).

Relationship to Culture and Religion

Medical procedures are inherently complex and difficult to understand. Patients and families must be able to comprehend the benefits and risks of procedures they consent to. Explicit explanation is especially important for patients and families who do not speak English as their primary language. An institution must have interpreters on hand to translate when informed consent is being obtained.

Case Example

A six-year-old Brazilian girl was to be admitted for cardiac surgery. Both her parents spoke conversational English, but a pre-admission telephone assessment identified Portuguese as their primary language. Although no Portuguese interpreters were on staff, arrangements were made to have a consultant-interpreter on-site when the family came to the admitting department. The interpreter was assigned to the case throughout the hospital stay. On the day of admission, the surgeon's detailed explanation of the surgery was translated by the interpreter. The parents stated they understood the risks and benefits and consented to the surgery. Later that day, the interpreter translated as a nurse oriented the family to the intensive care unit. The father began asking questions about the surgery and seemed confused about the details. The nurse paged one of the residents on the team and, through the interpreter, he explained the surgery once again. The parents were encouraged to write down questions as they arose for clarification later.

Comments

Medical procedures are often difficult for the lay person to understand. Several explanations may be necessary. In this scenario, although the parents had already consented to the surgery, they were given other opportunities for questions.

Sample Medical Record Documentation

Entry 1: "Six-year-old girl from Brazil admitted for repair of a ventricular septal defect. Both parents speak some English but state that they do not understand medical terminology in English. Consultant-interpreter scheduled for pre-admission clinic visit. During clinic visit, Dr. Z explained the surgery in detail through the interpreter. Parents state they understand the risks and benefits of the surgery and signed consent."

Entry 2: "Family oriented to intensive care unit with Portuguese interpreter translating. Father asking questions about bypass and the surgery tomorrow. Surgical procedure reviewed by nurse. Resident paged. Dr. T answered all questions regarding surgery. Parents encouraged to write down questions for medical team."

Patient Rights

Standard RI.1.2.2: "The family participates in care decisions" (Joint Commission, 1998, p. 50).

Relationship to Culture and Religion

Family roles and relationships differ from culture to culture and family to family. Even the definition of family has changed in recent years. A family member is anyone who plays a significant role in a person's life. This person may or may not be legally related. Family constellations are highly variable today with single parent families, foster families, gay or lesbian parents, and grandparents as primary caretakers. In some situations, the extended family is very involved in decision making. In others, involvement may be specific to a person's role in the family. Health care providers must respect all family members and include them in decision making as appropriate.

Case Example

The critically ill newborn infant of a lesbian mother was emergently transferred from the hospital of birth to a newborn intensive care unit (NICU) in a neighboring institution. The mother's partner and nonlegal parent of this newborn went to the NICU to visit the infant and check on her condition. Upon arrival to the unit, the nonlegal parent was denied visitation by the secretary who quoted the rules, "Parents only." The chaplain noticed this distraught woman in the hallway and offered to help. Once the chaplain was apprised of the situation, she advised the nurse, who put in a call to the birth mother. The birth mother was asked to identify the family members who would have permission to visit. She named her partner as the nonlegal parent and informed the nurse that they were intending to co-adopt the child. She then gave consent for her partner to visit and asked that she be involved in decisions regarding the infant's care.

Comment

Many nontraditional families exist in today's society, and providers must take care to avoid making assumptions. Establishing who is a family member and able to be involved in decisions is an important aspect of care (Earle, 1998). Simple, nonjudgmental questions can elicit this information and avoid undue stress. (See the section of the Introduction entitled Strategies for Providers on page xxiv.)

Sample Medical Record Documentation

"Infant admitted emergently to NICU with sepsis. Birth mother still at ABC hospital. Birth mother has a same-sex partner who is the nonlegal parent of infant. Birth mother gave telephone consent for nonlegal parent to visit and be involved in decisions regarding care. Consent for surgery or other procedures must be obtained from the birth mother at this time."

Standard RI.1.2.3, Standard RI.1.2.5, and Standard RI.1.2.6: "Patients are involved in resolving dilemmas about care decisions" (Joint Commission, 1998, p. 50); "The hospital addresses withholding resuscitative services" (Joint Commission, 1998, p. 51); "The hospital addresses foregoing or withdrawing life-sustaining treatment" (Joint Commission, 1998, p. 51).

Relationship to Culture and Religion

Decisions about care can be difficult when they involve withholding or withdrawing treatment. The cultural and religious values of patients and families may have an impact on these decisions. Organizations must have processes in place to help families address these issues with sensitivity (Joint Commission, 1998).

Case Example

A fifteen-year-old adolescent boy was admitted comatose and unresponsive to the medical intensive care unit (MICU) after ingesting an overdose of sedatives. In the course of the admission assessment, the nurse identified the patient and family as practicing Roman Catholics. She offered to call the hospital chaplain, and the family agreed. During her spiritual assessment, the chaplain learned that the patient and family were very involved in their local parish church. With the family's consent, the chaplain met with the parish priest, and the two clergy developed a plan of support for the family.

The patient's condition stabilized, but neurological tests determined that he was in a persistent vegetative state. Although he was breathing spontaneously, he required parenteral fluids and nutrition. The family began struggling with the ethical dilemma of whether to continue intravenous (IV) fluids and nutrition. The parents looked to the medical team and their parish priest for direction, and the parish priest sought expert theological consultation from authorities outside the local parish structure.

At this point the medical team asked for a consultation with the hospital's biomedical ethics committee. The family and parish priest joined the Ethics Advisory Committee meeting to discuss the discontinuation of nutrition and hydration. The group reviewed the ethical issues and discussed the patient's wishes. Finally, with the support of their priest, and in accordance with ethical and legal guidelines regarding the withdrawal of fluids and nutrients, the parents requested that IV fluids and nutrition be withdrawn. The patient died comfortably three days later. He remained in the ICU, although he no longer required critical care, because of the relationships that had been formed with the staff (Thiel & Robinson, 1997).

Comments

The hospital has a process for resolving ethical dilemmas, such as withholding or withdrawing life support. The Ethics Advisory Committee, a multidisciplinary team, aided the family in resolving this ethical dilemma. The parish priest was included as a team member because of the parents' strong faith and reliance on him as a spiritual advisor.

Sample Medical Record Documentation

"Neurological tests confirm persistent vegetative state (see neuro consult). Ethics consult called to assist parents in deciding whether parenteral nutrition and fluids will be withdrawn. Members of Ethics Advisory Committee met with family members and their parish priest. They discussed the patient's prognosis, patient's wishes, and the priest's explanation of the Catholic Church's teachings. With the support of the committee and their priest, the family decided to withdraw support. Patient will remain in the ICU."

Standard RI.1.2.7: "The hospital addresses care at the end of life" (Joint Commission, 1998, p. 52).

Relationship to Culture and Religion

Most cultures and religions follow bereavement rituals. The Joint Commission (1998) proposes that dying patients and their families need sensitive and respectful care that allows for expression of cultural and religious beliefs.

Case Example

A twelve-year-old girl had multiple critical injuries following a motor vehicle accident. Her condition was worsening, and the family was preparing for her impending death. All family members were involved in their Pentecostal church. In this religious tradition, dying persons are anointed by the elders of the church community. The family desired this for their daughter and requested permission to hold the ceremony in the intensive care unit. Despite the fact that there were fifteen elders plus family members, the staff in the ICU honored this family's need for a particular religious ritual by adapting the visitation rules. They moved the child to an isolation room for privacy during the service. The family and church elders sang hymns and anointed the young girl, and shortly thereafter she expired.

Comments

Although this service was potentially disruptive to the daily operations in the ICU, the staff recognized the need to accommodate the family's request. Bereavement rituals help families to grieve, and religious traditions are usually a source of comfort for those in mourning.

Sample Medical Record Documentation

"Patient on maximum ventilatory and vasopressor support. Dr. B spoke with the family and informed them that death was impending. Family requested that their daughter be anointed by the elders of their Pentecostal church. Patient moved into isolation room for privacy. Fifteen church members came to ICU and performed the anointing with the family in attendance. Patient expired at 8:05 p.m."

Standard RI.1.3: "The hospital demonstrates respect for the following patient needs: (RI.1.3.1) confidentiality; (RI.1.3.2) privacy; (RI.1.3.5) pastoral counseling; and (RI.1.3.6) communication."

Relationship to Culture and Religion

Most cultures have norms for confidentiality, privacy, and communication. Health care providers must be knowledgeable about family structures, relationships, and communication flow. For example, it may be important to include extended family members in certain discussions. In other families, parents may not want confidential information shared with the patient, such as a diagnosis of cancer. Use of eye contact, personal space norms, and the need for privacy are influenced by culture (Stewart, 1994). These issues must be taken into consideration when planning care. For patients with certain religious beliefs, pastoral counseling is an essential part of care and healing. The hospital must be able to provide for the needs of patients of all religious beliefs.

Case Example

A one-year-old Haitian boy was admitted to a medical unit with a diagnosis of HIV. The mother spoke Creole, and an interpreter was called. When the interpreter arrived, the mother became very upset and would not talk. The interpreter recognized the mother as a member of her church community and surmised that the mother was concerned with privacy, highly valued by many Haitians. Another interpreter, who did not know the mother, was called. The mother revealed that she did not want any family members or friends to know the diagnosis. She revealed that in Haiti, there is a strong stigma associated with the diagnosis of HIV, and she did not want her son to be the victim of prejudice. The staff respected the mother's wishes for confidentiality throughout the hospital stay.

Comments

Haitians are generally private people and may not disclose necessary information (Colin & Paperwala, 1996). Using the first interpreter who was assigned would have negatively affected the relationship of the health care team with the mother. Recognizing this mother's need for privacy constituted sensitive and respectful care.

Sample Medical Record Documentation

"Haitian mother of one-year-old requests confidentiality regarding patient diagnosis with all family members and friends. Use only G. Colin as interpreter (beeper #0000)."

Standard RI.2: "The hospital has a policy and procedures, developed with the medical staff's participation, for the procuring and donation of organs and other tissues" (Joint Commission, 1998, p. 54).

Relationship to Culture and Religion

Some religious traditions do not support organ donation. Providers need to be sensitive to families' beliefs regarding organ donation. Discretion must be used when asking families about organ donation.

Case Example

A ten-year-old girl was declared brain dead following a motor vehicle crash. She and her family were Greek Orthodox. Organ transplantation and donation are uncommon in this religious tradition because many believe that the body is sacred and should be buried with all its organs intact. (See Chapter 10 on Eastern Orthodox traditions.) The issue of organ donation was explored gently by the chaplain during a spiritual assessment, and the family declined. Although clinically the girl was a candidate for organ donation, the family was not approached again for organ and tissue donation.

Comments

The issue of organ donation is a very sensitive one. The health care team in this situation used discretion and did not cause undue emotional stress to the family.

Sample Medical Record Documentation

"Ten-year-old girl with irreversible brain damage (see neuro consult) is possible candidate for organ donation. Chaplain reports that family members are Greek Orthodox and have declined organ donation for religious reasons."

Standards Update, 2001

The following 2001 Joint Commission Standards have cultural and religious implications.

Patient Rights

Standard RI.1.2.7:"The health care organization addresses care at the end of life" (Joint Commission, 2001, p. 76).

Relationship to Culture and Religion

Dying patients have unique needs for care at the end of life. Just as culture and religion influence a patient's and family's response to illness and treatment, these two factors play a vital role in their understanding of dying and the days surrounding death. Health care providers are encouraged to explore the specific needs of the patient and family during the patient's final stages. Care at the end of life includes respect for these needs.

A Muslim man was dying in a local hospital. He was surrounded by family and friends. In the hours following his death, the family, although visibly grieving, was growing noticeably anxious and resistant to leaving the bedside. The medical staff was intent on removing the body from the floor and preparing it for post-mortem care. One of the family members asked what was going to happen to the patient now that he had died. The nurse called the Imam (Muslim chaplain) for consultation. After talking with the Imam and the family, the medical staff was able to attend to the patient's and family's requests—that the patient's body be cared for by a member of the same sex and religion, that his body be clothed at all times according to their specifications, and that the process be carried out with the patient facing East (toward Mecca).

Comments

Health care providers need to explore religious and cultural specifications surrounding post-mortem care. These important conversations should take place with the patient and family before death and also with clergy or spiritual leaders.

Sample Medical Record Documentation

"Patient is from Saudi Arabia. The patient and family are Muslim. They request the following: post-mortem care by a male technician of Muslim faith (non-Muslim may assist if wearing gloves); clothed at all times during preparation, head facing East and arms placed at his side."

Patient Rights

Standard RI.1.2.8: "Patients have the right to appropriate assessment and management of pain" (Joint Commission, 2001, p. 76)

Assessment of Patients

Standard PE.1.4: "Pain is assessed in all patients" (Joint Commission, 2001, p. 88).

Patient and Family Education

Standard PF.3.4: "Patients are educated about pain and managing pain as part of treatment, as appropriate" (Joint Commission, 2001, p. 134).

Relationship to Culture and Religion

Pain is often part of a patient's illness. It is essential for health care providers to respect the rights of all patients around pain management. Patients of different cultures and religions may be either unaccustomed to expressing and attending to their needs or more expressive than care givers are accustomed to. Health care providers are responsible for talking with patients and families about their roles in managing pain. Particularly when a caregiver and a patient speak different languages, it is essential to work with a trained interpreter who not only speaks the same language as the patient but also may understand the cultural nuances around pain.

Case Example One

A Chinese woman was admitted to a local hospital for extensive surgery. Following the operation, the nurse asked the patient how she felt, using a pain scale. The nurse asked the patient to point to the facial expression that best described her level of pain. The patient pointed to the drawing of a smiling face. Assuming that the patient was not in pain, the nurse left without administering the PRN pain medication. Later, the nurse noticed that the patient refused to get out of bed as instructed and was grimacing as if in pain. The patient's family was concerned that she was not well. Using an interpreter, the nurse talked with the patient and family about the use of pain medication and its importance in the recovery process. The nurse learned that the patient had used acupuncture in the past for pain management and at the family's request agreed to investigate how to arrange for the assistance of an acupuncturist. The patient agreed to try one dose of morphine 10 mg IV and had good results—pain relief without a change in consciousness.

Comments

Chinese patients may not verbalize their complaints, out of respect for others. They may also refuse pain medication because some believe that it impairs consciousness. Health care providers should explore with patients the use of pain therapies, both traditional and non-traditional, as a means to improve the recovery process.

Sample Medical Record Documentation

"Patient does not complain of pain but is grimacing upon movement. Patient points to smiling face but appears to be in pain. Interpreter called and RN discussed role of pain management in recovery process. Patient agreed to try one dose of morphine. 10mg morphine given IV with good results. Patient stated she felt comfortable and was not too sleepy. Daughter wishes to bring in family acupuncturist. RN will consult with supervisor as to how to arrange."

Case Example Two

A nurse, raised and trained in the New England area, was overheard commenting on her patient's pain-related complaints. The patient, a recent immigrant from Europe, was very expressive and vocal about the degree of pain she was feeling. The nurse seemed to be agitated by the "complaining." Upon further exploration, the nurse realized that her own upbringing was a factor in her response. She had been raised in a family in which pain was often overlooked and perhaps under-treated ("the stiff upper lip mentality," she called it). Her response to her patient, who was of a culture very comfortable with the expression of pain and grief, was a result of her own socialization.

Comments

Pain is an individual experience and should be treated as such. Health care providers need to be encouraged to explore their own feelings toward the treatment of pain and how these feelings may reflect on the care of patients so that they can respond in ways consistent with cultural competence.

Sample Medical Record Documentation

"Patient expresses increased pain today in lower lumbar area. When asked to quantify, through a Greek interpreter, her pain is a 7/10 (yesterday 5/10). See attached pain scale, circled by patient."

Ongoing Challenges

The intent of these standards is to ensure that patients receive care that is appropriate and congruent with their belief systems. If a provider recommends a medication or treatment that violates a patient's beliefs, the patient or family will most likely ignore the advice, jeopardizing his or her health status. Working within a patient's cultural and religious belief systems can help to increase understanding and treatment compliance. A critical step in this process is asking the right questions (see Strategies for Providers in the Introduction to this book) and performing a thorough patient assessment, the foundation for a culturally sensitive plan of care. Stewart (1994) notes that patient education is more effective when a patient's and family's cultural and religious beliefs are recognized, valued, and integrated into the teaching plan.

Although no clinician would argue with the good sense of these standards, they present a challenge. Many providers find it difficult to meet the standards for several reasons: difficulty with communication, unfamiliarity with many cultures and religions, discomfort with asking questions regarding a patient's religion and culture, time constraints, and lack of knowledge about the most effective way to document cultural and religious information (Murphy & Clark, 1993).

Earle (1998) argues that patients are usually pleased by the interest a provider shows about their cultural and religious customs. The key is to ask questions in a sensitive and diplomatic manner. These techniques are not necessarily intuitive, and training is essential. Staff training, using case examples, can be very helpful in developing cultural competence. Training cannot be a one-time event. It must be continuously integrated into the daily operations of patient care. Resources, such as this book, can also give providers a quick reference on the cultural and religious information they need.

References

Colin, J. M., & Paperwala, G. (1996). Haitians. In J. G. Lipson, S. L. Dibble, & P. A. Minarik (Eds.), *Culture and care: A pocket guide*. San Francisco: University of California San Francisco Nursing Press.

Cornett, S. J. (1993). Designing and implementing an effective patient education documentation system. In B. E. Gilroth (Ed.), *Managing hospital-based patient education*. Chicago, IL: American Hospital Publishing.

Earle, M., Jr. (1998, March). *Cultural implications in the care of the sick child*. Lecture presented at University of Massachusetts Children's Medical Center conference, Worcester, MA.

Joint Commission on Accreditation of Healthcare Organizations. (1998). *1998 Hospital accreditation standards*. Oakbrook Terrace, IL: JCAHO.

Lang, S. S. (1992). Understanding Hispanic diets. *Human Ecology Forum, 20*, 6–10.

Murphy, K., & Clark, J. M. (1993). Nurses' experiences in caring for ethnic-minority clients. *Journal of Advanced Nursing, 18*, 442–450.

Narayan, M. C. (1997). Cultural assessment in home healthcare. *Home Healthcare Nurse, 15*(10), 663–670.

Samolsky, S., Dunker, K., & Hynak-Hankinson, M. T. (1990). Feeding the Hispanic hospital patient: Cultural considerations. *Journal of the American Dietetic Association, 90*(12), 1707–1710.

Shiba, G., & Oka, R. (1996). Japanese Americans. In J. G. Lipson, S. L. Dibble, & P. A. Minarik (Eds.), *Culture and care: A pocket guide*. San Francisco: University of California San Francisco Nursing Press.

Stewart, B. (1994). Teaching culturally diverse populations. *Seminars in*

Perioperative Nursing, 3(3), 160–167.

Sumner, C. H. (1998). Recognizing and responding to spiritual distress. *American Journal of Nursing, 98*(1), 26–31.

Thiel, M. M., & Robinson, M. R. (1997). Physicians' collaboration with chaplains: Difficulties and benefits. *Journal of Clinical Ethics, 8*(1), 94–103.

Appendix

Standard for Nursing Practice: Culture and Care

Introduction

Culture refers to a set of values, beliefs, customs, and behaviors that connect a group of people. Culture influences beliefs about what causes illness and how it should be treated. These beliefs may guide patients' actions in health maintenance and illness. Understanding cultural perspectives can help the nurse appreciate why families may make certain decisions. As important as cultural norms may be, they do not necessarily predict the beliefs of an individual.

Need   To integrate cultural beliefs and practices into the patient/family's plan of care

Outcome Criteria   The child/family will have nursing care that incorporates their cultural needs as part of a holistic approach to health care.

Process Criteria

1. Establish a care team. Include interpreters whenever possible.

2. Acknowledge own (caregiver's) personal culture and beliefs.

3. Become acquainted with the cultural background of patients and family.

4. Provide for an interpreter for non-English speaking patients and their families upon admission and throughout the hospital course. The interpreter should have knowledge of the patient's and family's culture. Whenever possible, meet with the interpreter beforehand to plan for the patient interview.

5. When working with non-English speaking families, do not use family members or other patients or their families to elicit or convey information that is the basis for medical decisions.

6. Assess the patient's and family's comprehension of the child's illness.

7. Recognize those patients' and families' values and beliefs that will affect their learning process and integration of new ideas.

8. Establish outcome expectations mutually with the patient and family, incorporating cultural needs and values into the plan of care.

9. Individualize the teaching plan using effective teaching methods such as written handouts, videos, or demonstrations. Utilize verbal and written translated teaching materials for non-English speaking patients and families.

10. Avoid stereotyping and imposing expectations on the basis of personal standards, attitudes, and beliefs.

11. Utilize hospital resources on the cultural aspects of care, such as interpreter services and cultural consultants.

12. Document the assessment, plan, interventions, and evaluation of teaching incorporating cultural information.

Rationale Knowledge of cultural beliefs and values is essential in practicing holistic care. Understanding the child and family from their cultural perspective will enhance care provided and diminish the potential for misunderstandings.

References

Ahmann, E. (1994, May–June). Chunky stew: Appreciating cultural diversity while providing health care for children. *Pediatric Nursing, 20*(3), 320–323.

Buchwald, D., Caralis, P. V., Gany, F., Hardt, E., Johnson, T. M., Muecke, M., & Putsche, R. (1994, June 15). Caring for patients in a multicultural society. *Patient Care*, pp. 104–123.

Kinsman, S., Mitchell, S., & Fox, K. (1996, October). Multicultural issues in pediatric practice. *Pediatrics in Review, 17*(10), 349–354.

Kleinman, A., Eisenberg, L., & Good, B. (1978, February). Culture, illness, and care: Clinical lessons from anthropologic and cross-cultural research. *Annals of Internal Medicine, 88*(2), 251–260.

Price, J. L., & Cordell, B. (1994, August). Cultural diversity and patient teaching. *Journal of Continuing Education in Nursing, 25*(4), 163–166.

Emergency Baptism Procedures

Policy

It is the policy of the Department of Pastoral Care to make available the sacrament of baptism to Christian patients in times of medical emergency. In cases other than medical emergency or special necessity, baptism shall be celebrated in the patient's church community.

Guidelines

Emergencies are typically understood as situations in which a child's life is perceived by a parent or staff as in danger. Routine baptisms are not typically performed in the hospital setting. The religion of the patient as stated by the competent patient, parent, or legal guardian shall determine the appropriate procedure.

Emergency Baptism of Roman Catholic Patients

1. Roman Catholic tradition requires unbaptized children to be baptized immediately if their lives are in jeopardy.

2. The child's baptismal status can be found on the front sheet of the chart (CAY = baptized, CAN = not baptized). Whenever possible, staff shall consult with the parents or guardian prior to baptizing.

3. To request an emergency baptism, staff shall contact the Catholic chaplain assigned to the unit or on call via the switchboard. Normally, the Catholic chaplain will baptize. If the Catholic chaplain on call is unavailable or cannot arrive in time, anyone may baptize. (See Procedure for Baptism on following page.)

Emergency Baptism of Protestant Patients

1. Protestant tradition varies in its requirement for emergency baptism. (Some churches do not baptize at all; others baptize adults only.) In the event of a medical emergency, nursing or medical staff shall speak with the parents or guardians to ascertain their desire for baptism.

2. To request an emergency baptism, staff shall contact the Catholic chaplain assigned to the unit or on-call via the switchboard. Normally, the Catholic chaplain will baptize. If the Catholic chaplain

on call is unavailable or cannot arrive in time, anyone may baptize. (See Procedure for Baptism below.)

Procedure for Baptism

The person baptizing will pour water on the forehead (if the forehead is not possible, on any flesh available), in such a way that it will flow on the skin. While the water is being poured, the person baptizing shall say, audibly, "I baptize you in the name of the Father, and of the Son, and of the Holy Spirit. Amen."

Retain the following information: child's name, date and place of birth, maiden name of mother, name of father, name of person baptizing, witnesses, date of baptism. That information shall be forwarded to the Department of Pastoral Care.

Prepare a baptismal certificate, proofread it, and give it to the family or guardian at the time of baptism.

Chaplains on staff at Children's shall chart the baptism in the progress notes of the patient's medical record. On-call clergy shall provide and fill out a sticker for addition to the progress note.

The Department of Pastoral Care shall maintain a Baptismal Log as a permanent record of all baptisms taking place within the hospital.

Catholic baptisms must also be recorded at Mission Church, Tremont Street, Boston.

Ethics Committee Consultation

An informal discussion about ethical dimensions of a patient care situation may be obtained by calling the Ethics Advisory Committee co-chairs, paging the operator, or by talking with past or present members of the committee.

A formal ethics consultation of the Ethics Advisory Committee can be initiated by any member of the care team, the patient, or the family as follows:

1. When a morally troubling or complex problem occurs, the usual processes are discussion by immediately involved caregivers; an interdisciplinary care conference; and meeting with family, significant others, and their close advisors, such as a religious counselor or family advocate.

2. If this standard procedure results in disagreement or the desire to further explore the ethical aspects of decisions, a member of the care team or the family can consult the EAC through one of the co-chairs as described above.

3. A committee co-chair or designated committee member will meet with the consultee to learn more about the problem and the kind of advice caregivers need from the EAC. A decision will be made whether to initiate a formal consultation. Other resources in the hospital may be suggested to provide help, for example, a chaplain or someone from Social Work or Patient Relations.

4. The caregiver(s) and/or family should then prepare a brief written synopsis of the case history, present situation, and prognosis and identify the ethical question(s) about which they seek advice.

5. A meeting of an ethics consulting team or the full EAC will be scheduled (usually within twenty-four hours). Notification, calling, and scheduling will be done through the office of the administrative representative to the committee.

6. The attending physician, primary nurse, and other caregivers from the various disciplines who are directly involved in and knowledgeable about the care of the patient and family should be notified by the consultee and invited to attend the consultation meeting.

---

7. The family should be informed by the attending physician, consultee, or designated team member that the EAC has been consulted and will be meeting to discuss the case. The family should be invited to meet with the EAC meeting if they desire. There is no requirement that the family meet with the EAC. There is, however, an expectation that the family will be offered the opportunity to do so either in the consulting session or separately.

8. The EAC and caregivers or family meet together to discuss the case and their ethical concerns. The consultee, the attending physician, and others present are invited to give their input. The ethical question(s) to be addressed are identified.

9. Input from the meeting with the family may be added, if already obtained, or the family may meet with EAC members then or later.

10. The EAC in executive session discusses and may elaborate on the ethical question(s), analyzes the problem, applies ethical principles and reasoning, and explores morally permissible alternatives for resolution.

11. The committee's deliberations and advice are communicated verbally to the consultee and other available team members immediately following the end of the meeting, and a summary of same is written in the Progress Notes of the patient's medical record by one of the committee co-chairs or designated committee member. The consultee or attending physician is responsible for communicating the results of the ethics consultation to the family as appropriate. The family may have a copy of the consultation.

12. The EAC will usually provide a more thorough and detailed analysis of the ethical question(s) raised by the consultation, the committee's moral reasoning, and their advice within ten days—to be available to caregivers and interested others as an educational tool. This document does not become part of the patient's permanent record, but may be shared with family.

Ethics of Redirecting Goals of Care

Introduction

Children's Hospital is committed to restoring health and sustaining life in the patients it serves. There are instances, however, when certain medical interventions may no longer prove to be in the patient's best interest. For some patients, it may be appropriate to change the goals of treatment from a focus on cure to a focus on comfort. The purpose of this document is to address ethical considerations and provide guidelines for caregivers involved in decisions related to redirecting the goals of care.

Statement of General Principles

1. Open and timely communication among the patient, family, and members of the health care team is central to optimal ethical decision making.

2. Parents are the decision makers for minor patients, unless they clearly act against their child's best interest or are unable, unwilling, or persistently unavailable to make decisions on behalf of their child.

3. Pediatric patients who have attained a sufficient cognitive and developmental level to understand and evaluate their treatment options should generally be given substantial consideration in the decision-making process.

4. Competent adult patients may designate a proxy or surrogate to make all medical decisions on their behalf should they become incapacitated. For information on advance directives and the Patient Self-Determination Act, caregivers should contact the Office of General Counsel.

5. A redirection to comfort-focused care is a change of goals, not a withdrawal of care, concern, or intervention.

6. The duty of health professionals to promote the health and well-being of their patients does not entail an absolute duty to preserve life by all means. For example, it is ethically permissible to limit life-sustaining treatment when it is refused by a patient who is a competent adult. In addition, life-sustaining treatment may be limited in the care of children and incompetent parents when the health care

team and the parents or surrogate agree that such treatment is not in the patient's best interest.

7. There is no ethical obligation to provide life-sustaining treatment when its use is not consistent with the goals of the patient's treatment plan, nor when the clinical team believes that the benefit of treatment no longer outweighs the burdens. Disagreement about these obligations should never be resolved unilaterally, however, but should be processed through mechanisms that are available to promote optimal decision making in situations of conflict (for example, clinical team meetings, interventions from Social Work and Pastoral Care, consultations from the Ethics Advisory Committee, or advice from the Office of General Counsel).

8. In contemporary bioethics, there is no ethically significant difference between withdrawing (stopping) and withholding (not starting) life-sustaining treatment.

9. A variety of medical treatments may be considered life sustaining, depending on the patient's condition. These may range from renal dialysis and mechanical ventilation to antibiotics and tube feedings. Under appropriate circumstances, all medical treatment may be withheld or withdrawn, except procedures for alleviating pain or promoting comfort. Artificial nutrition and hydration (that is, tube feedings and parenteral nutrition) are forms of medical treatment and their use or discontinuation should be governed by the same medical and ethical considerations as for other forms of life-sustaining treatment.

11. There are important ethical distinctions between letting a patient die and euthanasia. In letting a patient die, the cause of death is the underlying disease process or trauma. In euthanasia, the cause of death may be defined as the intended lethal action.

12. The use of medications and other interventions that may potentially hasten death may be ethically justifiable when they are used with the intent of relieving suffering, but is not justifiable when they are used with the intent of causing the patient's death. In addition, the benefits of providing pain relief must outweigh the harm or risk of potentially hastening death, and these medications and interventions must be used only when there are not any less harmful treatments that could also be effective at relieving the patient's pain and suffering.

13. Resort to judicial intervention by the hospital should occur only when unresolvable conflicts remain between the care team and the family or among the care team itself, and only after good faith efforts have been made to achieve consensus. The Office of General Counsel has the responsibility of deciding when or whether judicial intervention is appropriate.

Guidelines for Redirecting Goals of Care

Patient Identification   Redirection of the goals of care should be considered for any patient when the benefits of continued attempts to achieve a cure or prolong life no longer exceed the burdens imposed by those attempts. This assessment must always be made from the perspective of the patient, and must never be based on a perception of the patient's "social worth." In most cases, redirection of the goals of care will arise in the context of a terminal illness or condition. In some cases, however, the availability and use of sophisticated life-sustaining interventions may confound the ability of caregivers (and family members) to perceive a patient as "terminally ill" or "dying." In other cases (for example, a patient in a persistent vegetative state), redirection of the goals of care may be justified, even though the patient may not be terminally ill. Rather than focusing on whether or not a patient is dying, therefore, ethical analysis should focus on the balance between the benefits and burdens of continued therapy, as viewed from the perspective of the patient.

In addition, because the perception of the benefits and burdens of therapy will vary between individuals and families, based on their experiences and values, patients with similar clinical conditions may request different goals of treatment. Two patients with identical stages of an advanced malignancy, for example, may reasonably choose different goals, with one focusing on cure and the other focusing on comfort.

Discussion Between Health Care Team and Family   Open and thorough discussion between the family and the health care team is essential in order to provide optimal patient care and to show respect for the moral and religious sensibilities of those involved. Children and adolescents should generally be informed and involved in discussions about their diagnosis, prognosis, and treatment options, in a manner commensurate with their ability to comprehend and tolerate the information.

In general, discussions about the appropriate use of medical interventions and life-sustaining treatment should be an ongoing process, not a simple one-time urgent event. Such discussions are optimally undertaken within the context of an established family-caregiver relationship. Therefore, it is important that the primary doctor and primary nurse coordinate regularly scheduled family meetings to address the patient's condition, the response to treatment, and the plan of care.

Any member of the health care team, the patient, or the family may initiate discussion about the appropriateness of life-sustaining treatment and the possible redirection of care. It is the responsibility of the primary doctor and the primary nurse to facilitate discussion of the overall goals of patient care, as well as to evaluate whether the treatments provided are congruent with those goals of patient care. Again, it should be emphasized that a redirection to comfort-focused care is a change of goals, not a withdrawal of care.

Decision-Making Procedures   Decision making about life-sustaining treatment is considered a shared responsibility between the health care team and the family, which is consistent with Children's Hospital philosophy of family-centered patient care. In general, parents have the responsibility to make health care decisions for their minor children. Adult patients have the responsibility to make their own decisions regarding life-sustaining treatments unless they are deemed incompetent to do so. Children and adolescents who have attained a sufficient cognitive and developmental level to understand and evaluate their treatment options would generally be given substantial consideration in the decision-making process.

Physicians, nurses, and other health care professionals should anticipate clinical and ethical decision points (for example, tracheostomy, dialysis, DNR orders, and so forth) and provide families with as much time as possible to deliberate about their treatment options and moral choices. If it is unlikely that the patient can improve or survive, this information should be conveyed to the family, along with the option of redirecting the goals of care from a focus on cure to a focus on comfort. It is important that the primary caregivers provide not only clinical information, but also professional advice and guidance about how to best meet the patient's needs. The caregivers should seek input from the patient and family on their personal values and feelings about the short-term and long-term goals for the patient. The family should not, however, be put in the position of feeling that they have the sole responsibility of deciding whether or not their child should live or die. They should be told that the course of the disease is dictating a narrow range of options and that the health care team will share responsibility in deciding which of these options best meets the needs of the patient. In addition, families should be reassured that their child would not be abandoned. The family should be told that the health care team will work as hard at providing comfort as they did to provide cure.

In this decision-making process, there often has been an inappropriate emphasis on the simple duality of "DNR" or "non-DNR" status. The decision to not resuscitate a patient in the event of a cardiac arrest is but one component of defining the intensity of care. Although not every scenario can be anticipated in advance, decisions should be made about whether major interventions (for example, mechanical ventilation, chest tubes, vasoactive infusions, and so forth) should be initiated, continued, or withdrawn. The hospital's "DNR Order Sheet" requires explicit decisions concerning these interventions. The guiding principle is to ensure that all therapies are consistent with the goals of care.

The primary physician and the primary nurse should write a note summarizing each discussion with the family and delineating the management plan in the patient's chart. This note should be as specific as possible to ensure consistency of care delivery.

Although the great majority of situations are handled without conflict between the patient, family, and caregivers, at times even the best of efforts will result in a failure to reach consensus around medical interventions and the goals of treatment. In these situations, the family and/or care team should be encouraged to consult the Ethics Advisory Committee in the hope that decision making will be facilitated.

Patient Management   Explicit verbal and written communication among the members of the health care team will facilitate consistent patient management.

However, treatment issues will inevitably arise that have not been previously addressed in a formal meeting. In situations in which a decision has been made to focus on the patient's comfort rather than cure, the axiom for determining whether or not a given therapy is suitable is, "Do what will make the patient more comfortable." The corollary is, "Avoid things that will make the patient more uncomfortable." Disagreement about what defines "comfort" should be anticipated. Some issues may not be clear. For example, the use of antibiotics to treat a pneumonia that is causing respiratory distress could be seen as a comfort measure by some and as an inappropriate life-prolonging measure by others. When there is disagreement or uncertainty related to these principles, a meeting between the family and team should be convened. In addition, changes in the patient's condition and/or prognosis may warrant new discussions. If there is conflict after input from all involved parties, a consultation from the Ethics Advisory Committee may facilitate the decision-making process.

Religious Objections to Blood Transfusions

General Guidelines

Minors   Courts have uniformly intervened to order hospitals to give blood transfusions to minors over the religious objections of their Jehovah's Witnesses' or Christian Scientist parents. Thus, if a minor requires blood and the parents object, you should contact the Office of General Counsel to obtain a court order authorizing the blood transfusion. In the event of an emergency, the blood can be administered while the Office of General Counsel is simultaneously being contacted.

Adults   An adult who is mentally competent may usually refuse a life-saving blood transfusion. If the patient is pregnant or there are minor children involved, however, the court may override the patient's objections and order the blood transfusion. Thus, if an adult requires blood and yet refuses to have it administered, the Office of General Counsel should be consulted as to whether a court order should be sought. If it is decided that a court order will not be sought, the Office of General Counsel will seek to have the patient sign a waiver releasing the hospital from any liability associated with not giving a blood transfusion.

Hospital Policy and Procedures Regarding Religious Objections

Informed Consent Process   Parents whose religions forbid blood transfusions should be informed that Children's Hospital will make every effort to avoid giving their child blood, but that if in order to save their child's life it becomes necessary to administer blood, the hospital will obtain an emergency order authorizing it to do so. No guarantees should be given to the parents that blood will not be transfused because the hospital will in fact obtain an emergency order to do so if a blood transfusion becomes necessary to save the child's life. Parents may be permitted to amend the general or operative consent form to reflect their refusal to consent to the transfusion of blood. It is suggested, however, that—in addition to allowing the parents to amend the consent form(s)—the following language should be adopted to reflect the hospital's policy:

> Children's Hospital will make every effort to avoid administering blood to your child; however, if in the opinion of your physician it becomes necessary to do so in order to save your child's life, a court order will be sought authorizing blood transfusion.

If, after discussing the possibility that blood may be given pursuant to a court order, the parents seek to discharge their child, the Office of General Counsel should be consulted. The hospital most likely would not oppose a discharge if the parents are admitting the child to another facility. However, if the parents decide against any treatment at all because of the possibility of a blood transfusion, the hospital may need to consider initiating a care and protection proceeding and obtain a telephone emergency order preventing the child's discharge.

Information Needed to Obtain a Court Order   In order to obtain a court order, the Office of General Counsel needs to present the following information to the court:

Patient's full name;

Patient's date of birth;

Parents' full names;

Patient's attending physician's name;

Medical procedure that was done or is to be done on the patient;

Current medical condition of patient, particularly in regard to the need for blood;

Efforts made not to give blood;

Probability of having to administer blood;

Patient's response when Children's Hospital requests permission to consent to blood transfusion;

Parents' response to their child's needs, apart from refusal to consent to blood transfusion; and

Estimate of how long an emergency order should remain in effect.

Thus it is important to have this information available if you contact the Office of General Counsel regarding obtaining a court order.

In addition, after obtaining a court order to administer blood, a hearing will be held at the hospital at which the physician involved will have to testify.

Organ and Tissue Donation

In compliance with Massachusetts General Law Chapter 360, Section 8b, it is the policy of Children's Hospital (the "Hospital") to offer families the opportunity to consider organ and/or tissue donation whenever a death occurs. The patient's next of kin or other specified individual shall be approached concerning donation when appropriate.

Implementation of this policy requires sensitivity to the family circumstances regarding potential donation. Compliance with this policy must be appropriately documented in all deceased patients' medical records in the progress notes and, when consent has been obtained, on the Consent for Organ and Tissues Donation Form.

Almost anyone who dies can be a donor. While organ donation requires the special circumstances of brain death, tissue donation is possible with very few exceptions. The hospital shall participate in the recovery of anatomical gifts in cooperation with the New England Organ Bank (NEOB), other tissue banks, and medical schools.

The New England Organ Bank staff is available 24 hours a day to provide the necessary assistance in all aspects of the donation process. Call 1-800-446-6362.

Procedure

In the event of expectant or actual death:

Brain Death Declared or Pending   Brain dead patients up to 70 years old can be considered for organ and/or tissue donation. Contact the New England Organ Bank regarding the patient's suitability for donation. Brain dead patients over age 70 can be considered for eye donation only.

Other Deceased Patients   All other deceased patients can be considered for tissue donation according to the hospital's published criteria. In general, patients up to age 55 can be considered for bone, heart valve, eye, and skin donation. Patients over age 55 can be considered for eye and skin donation. Patients over age 70 can be considered for eye donation only.

Contact the New England Organ Bank   Do not hesitate to call the NEOB at 1-800-446-6362 for assistance with any or all aspects of the organ and tissue donation procedure.

Document the Result   If organ or tissue donation is ruled out in consultation with NEOB staff or according to screening criteria, document this in the medical record progress notes.

Inform the Family   Notify the family of the patient's expected or actual death. The physician, according to Children's Hospital's Brain Death Protocol, does the declaration of brain death.

Determine the Team Member   Determine the most appropriate person to discuss the donation option with the next of kin. The health care team member, such as the physician, primary nurse, social worker, or clergy member, who has developed a rapport with the family of the potential donor can assume this responsibility. The transplant surgeon should not obtain consent. The Organ Bank staff is available twenty-four hours a day to participate in the consent process.

Give Options   Offer the next of kin the option of tissue and/or organ donation. This decision is one the family has the right to make. If donation is refused, document this in the medical record in progress notes and on the Report of Death form.

Obtain Consent   The Organ Bank staff is available to obtain written or telephone consent, or will contact tissue bank staff to provide the same. A health care team member who is comfortable with all aspects of the donation and informed consent processes may obtain written or telephone consent. Two witnesses are required. The next of kin's wishes will prevail in this situation, but the patient's previously expressed wishes should be considered in this discussion. The next of kin order of priority is as follows:

1. Spouse

2. Adult son or daughter

3. Either parent

4. Adult brother or sister

5. Guardian of the decedent at the time of death

6. Any person authorized or under any obligation to dispose of the body

In accordance with the legislation, families should not be approached for donation under the following circumstances:

1. Staff member has knowledge that the donor or person authorized to consent is opposed to organ and tissue donation;

2. The request will cause undue emotional stress to the family;

3. The organs and tissues would be unsuitable according to medical criteria defined by transplanting physicians, department of Public Health, or New England Organ Bank.

Any questions regarding consent should be directed to the Office of the General Counsel.

Obtain Release of the Donor's Body   Obtain release of the body from the medical examiner when necessary.

Participate in Donor Management with the Organ Bank Staff   Work with the organ bank as needed to assure successful completion.

Document   Provide necessary documentation in the medical record, as follows:

1. Declaration of Death, including date and time

2. Consent for Organ and Tissue Donation

3. Medical Examiner's Clearance and/or Restrictions, when indicated

Contact Appropriate Staff   In the event consent is granted for organ and/or bone donation, the operating room (OR) staff shall be contacted by either the nursing supervisor or organ bank coordinator. The patient's name, organs, and tissues to be recovered, timing of surgery, and procedural details must be relayed to the OR staff. The Organ Bank arranges for a transplant team to perform the procedure.

Determine Timing of Donation   Recovery of eye, skin, and heart for valves can be carried out in the morgue. Donation timing can be coordinated by the nursing supervisor or administrator on call in conjunction with the Organ and Tissue Bank staff.

Patient and Family Education

Introduction and Description

Through collaboration with the multidisciplinary health care team and family, the primary nurse (or delegate) is responsible for ensuring that patient and/or family learning needs are identified and addressed. Learning is facilitated through integration of knowledge, attitudes, and experiences. It is a cooperative effort between the teacher (nurse) and the learner (patient or family) and ultimately results in an observable change in skills, behavior, and attitudes.

Need: To Assess Patient and/or Family Learning Needs

Outcome Criteria   Patient and/or family learning needs regarding the health and treatment plan are identified.

Process Criteria

1. Begin assessment and identification of learning needs during the admission process or outpatient interview. Ask open-ended questions.

2. Identify the need for an interpreter.

3. Through collaboration with the patient and family, identify specific learning needs (for example, disease process and treatment plan, well child care, medications, diet, equipment, physical care, or additional resources).

4. Identify learners (for example, patient, family, significant other) for each assessed learning need; this may vary with the task.

5. Observe both verbal and nonverbal cues to determine readiness, motivation, and ability to learn (for example, eye contact, attentiveness, and expressed fear of the task to be learned).

6. Determine past experiences and current level of knowledge relating to the learning needs.

7. Identify individual learning style(s), comprehension level, and literacy when determining the most appropriate means to meet the identified learning need (for example, reading, hands-on demonstration, video, and puppetry).

8. Identify cultural, developmental, psychosocial, spiritual, and physical factors in considering the needs and ability to provide care. Recognize barriers to learning.

9. Assess socioeconomic influences (for example, finances, insurance, occupation) on learning needs and ability to provide care.

10. Identify the need for continuing support and education through community agencies and services (such as the Visiting Nurse Association) and the primary care provider.

Rationale   All patients come to the hospital with some learning needs. How learning is accomplished varies according to the individual and the task. The assessment process identifies needs and barriers to learning.

Need: To Plan the Learning Experience

Outcome Criteria   Incorporating assessed learning needs will result in the development of a dynamic patient/family teaching plan.

Process Criteria

1. Describe the teaching plan in the Patient Management Plan. Include in the teaching plan: realistic, measurable objectives, use of tools, and identification of both learners and teachers.

2. Plan time needed to meet learning objectives based on the patient's acuity, learning needs, and anticipated length of stay.

3. Document interventions to be completed by each member of the multidisciplinary team, for example, nurses, nurse specialists, physicians, social services, physical therapists, child life specialists, and nutritionists.

Rationale   Planning strategies based on the assessed learning needs will facilitate a cohesive, individualized learning experience.

Need: To Implement the Teaching Plan

Outcome Criteria   Learning will progress according to the individualized teaching plan.

Process Criteria

1. Utilize a multidisciplinary approach.

2. Provide for flexibility in the teaching process, adapting to changes in the learner's needs or patient's condition. Build on the learner's previous experience.

3. Set implementation priorities. Focus on what the learner needs to know versus what is nice to know, what the learner should do and why, when to expect results, possible danger signs, what to do if problems arise, and whom to contact.

4. Provide a learning environment conducive to the task at hand.

5. Address patient and family barriers to learning (pain, stress, literacy) and outstanding concerns.

6. Utilize opportunities for formal or informal teaching.

7. Use various teaching styles (lecture and demonstration) to meet learning objectives.

8. Provide teaching aids to facilitate learning (information sheets, videos, demonstration dolls).

9. Offer a clear rationale for each teaching step. Be specific and logical. Avoid medical jargon.

10. Restate critical information in various ways.

11. Provide adequate time for assimilation of information. Difficult tasks may take a longer period of time to grasp. The learner may need to have information repeated.

12. Involve community and outpatient services in the teaching process, as indicated. Provide appropriate referrals.

13. Document patient and family progress toward meeting learning objectives. Documentation should include what was taught, response to teaching, understanding of the material presented, and any alterations in the teaching plan.

Rationale   Learning outcomes are enhanced by utilization of a flexible and individualized teaching plan that, applied in a systemic manner, reflects patient and/or family learning needs and response to teaching.

Need: To Evaluate the Teaching Plan

Outcome Criteria   Learning needs have been met as evidenced by return demonstration of procedures and verbal comprehension.

Process Criteria

1. Through observation and verbal interaction, determine the effectiveness and learner's comprehension of each teaching step.

2. Document the teaching process to reflect the learner's understanding of the task or concept taught; the learner's proficiency in meeting

learning objectives and, if not met, why not; completion of the teaching and learning plan prior to patient discharge; and follow-up or continuity of the teaching plan to community providers when appropriate.

3. Revise the teaching plan or interventions as indicated by evaluation of the learning objectives.

Rationale   The process of patient and family education requires continuous assessment and evaluation of progress. Provide opportunity for restructuring of the plan as needed.

References

Katz. J. R . (1997, May). Back to basics: Providing effective patient teaching. *American Journal of Nursing*, (5), 33–36.

Lorig, K., Gonzalez, V., & Romer, L. (1996). *A guide to educating patients*. San Bruno, CA: Krames Communications.

Volker, D. L. (1991, January). Needs assessment and resource identification. *Oncology Nursing Forum, 18*(1), 119–123.

References and Other Resources

Books and Journals

Ahmann, E. (1994). Chunky stew: Appreciating cultural diversity while providing healthcare for children. *Pediatric Nursing, 20*(3), 320–324.

Bloom, M. (1996). The use of interpreters in interviewing: Characteristics, conceptualization and cautions. *Mental Hygiene, 50*(2) 214–17.

Botvin, G., Schinke, S., & Orlandi, M. (1995). *Drug abuse prevention with multiethnic youth.* Thousand Oaks, CA: Sage.

Buchwald, D., Caralis, P. V., Gany, F., Hardt, E., Johnson, T. M., & Muecke, M. (1994, June 15). Caring for patients in a multicultural society. *Patient Care,* pp. 105–123.

Bumer, O. Y., Cunningham, P., & Haftar, H. S. (1990). Managing a multicultural nurse staff in a multicultural environment. *Journal of Nursing Administration, 20*(6), 30–34.

Castex, G. M. (1994). Providing services to Hispanic/Latino populations: Profiles in diversity. *Journal of the NASW, 39*(3), 288–296.

Chin, J. L., De la Cancela, V., & Jenkins, Y. (1993). *Diversity and psychotherapy: The politics of race, ethnicity and gender.* Westport, CT: Praeger.

Council of Churches of Greater Springfield and the Visiting Nurse Hospice of Pioneer Valley. (1995). *Knowing my neighbor: Religious beliefs and cultural traditions at times of illness and death.* Springfield, MA: Council of Churches.

Culley, L. (1996). A critique of multiculturalism in healthcare: The challenge for nurse education. *Journal of Advanced Nursing, 23,* 564–570.

David Kennedy Center for International Studies. (1996). *Culturgrams: El Salvador, Guatemala, Honduras, India, Mexico, Puerto Rico, Saudi Arabia.* Provo, UT: Brigham Young University.

DeSantis, L. (1988). Cultural factors affecting newborn and infant diarrhea. *Journal of Pediatric Nursing, 3*(6), 391–398.

Eliason, M. J. (1993, September/October). Ethics and transcultural nursing care. *Nursing Outlook, 41,* 225–228.

Elyasberg, Y. (1996). *Voices of the Soviet Jewish community.* Seattle, WA: University of Washington: Healthlinks.

Eschleman, M. J. (1992, November). Death with dignity. *Today's O.R. Nurse,* pp. 19–23.

Fox, K. (1997, September 25). Inequities in health care closely correlated to race, income level. *Bay State Banner,* p. 9a.

Friedman, M. M. (1992). *Family nursing: Theory and practice* (3rd ed.). Norwalk, CT: Appleton & Lange.

Giger, J. N., & Davidhizar, R. E. (1995). *Transcultural nursing: Assessment and intervention* (2nd ed.). St. Louis, MO: Mosby.

Giger, J. N., Davidhizar, R. E., Parsons, L., & Holcomb, L. (1996). Haitian Americans: Implications for nursing care. *Journal of Community Health Nursing, 13*(4), 249–260.

Goldsby, B., & Smith, S. (1995). *Families in multicultural perspective.* New York: Guilford Press.

Gontron Lamberty, P. H., & Garcia Coll, C. (1994). *Puerto Rican women and children: Issues in health, growth and development.* New York: Plenum Press.

Green, N. L. (1995). Development of the perceptions of racism scale. *Image: Journal of Nursing Scholarship, 27*(2), 141–146.

Habayeb, G. L. (1995). Cultural diversity: A nursing concept not yet reliably defined. *Nursing Outlook, 43*(5), 224–227.

Hahn, M. S. (1995, November). Providing healthcare in a culturally complex world. *ADVANCE for Nurse Practitioners,* pp. 43–45.

Harwood, A. (1981). *Ethnicity and medical care.* Cambridge, MA: Harvard University Press.

Jones, E. G., & Kay, M. (1992). Instrumentation in cross-cultural research. *Nursing Research, 41*(3), 186–188.

Kinsman, S. B., Mitchell, S., & Fox, K. (1996, October). Multicultural issues in pediatric practice. *Pediatrics in Review, 17*(10), 349–355.

Kirkwood, N. (1995). *Hospital handbook on multiculturalism and religion.* Harrisburg, PA: Morehouse.

Kleinman, A., Eisenberg, L., & Good, B. (1978, February). Culture, illness, and care. *Annals of Internal Medicine, 88*(2), 251–258.

Lewis, T., Hussein, K., Ahmed, K., Ahmed, B., & Mohammed, A. (1996). Somali families. University of Washington, Healthlinks. *Ethnomed: www.hslib.washington.edu/clinical/ethnomed/somali.htm*

Lipson, J. G., Dibble, S. L., & Minarik, P. A. (Eds.). (1997). *Culture & nursing care: A pocket guide.* San Francisco: University of California San Francisco Nursing Press.

Luna, L. J. (1989, Summer). Transcultural nursing care of Arab Muslims. *Journal of Transcultural Nursing, 1*(1), 22–26.

Lynch, E. W., & Hanson, M. J. (Eds.). (1992). *Developing cross-cultural competence: A guide for working with young children and their families.* Baltimore, MD: Paul H. Brookes Publishing.

McGoldrick, M., Giordano, J., & Pearce, J. K. (Eds.). (1996). *Ethnicity and family therapy* (2nd ed.). New York: Guilford Press.

McIntosh, P. (1989, July/August). White privilege: Unpacking the white knapsack. *Peace and Freedom,* pp. 10–12.

Mitchell, P. R., & Grippando, G. M. (1993). *Nursing perspectives and issues* (5th ed.). Albany, NY: Delmar Publishers.

Molakign, A. (1996). Ethiopian families. University of Washington, Healthlinks. *Ethnomed: www.hslib.washington.edu/clinical/ethnomed/ethiopcp.htm*

Moorhead, G., & Griffin, R. W. (1995). *Organizational behavior* (4th ed.). Boston, MA: Houghton Mifflin.

Mulholland, J. (1995). Nursing, humanism and transcultural theory: The bracketing-out of reality. *Journal of Advanced Nursing, 22,* 442–449.

Noraidah bte Abdullah, S. (1995). Towards an individualized client's care: Implications for education. The transcultural approach. *Journal of Advanced Nursing, 22,* 715–720.

Office of Refugee and Immigrant Health. (1995). *Refugees and immigrants in Massachusetts fact sheets.* Boston, MA: Office of Multi-Cultural Services/ Refugee Assistance Program, Massachusetts Department of Public Health.

Park Ridge Center for the Study of Health, Faith, and Ethics. (1995). *The Jehovah's Witness tradition: Religious beliefs and health care decisions.* Chicago, IL: Park Ridge Center.

Park Ridge Center for the Study of Health, Faith, and Ethics. (1995). *The Jewish tradition: Religious beliefs and health care decisions.* Chicago, IL: Park Ridge Center.

Park Ridge Center for the Study of Health, Faith, and Ethics. (1995). *The Protestant tradition: Religious beliefs and health care decisions.* Chicago, IL: Park Ridge Center.

Peterson, R., & Smith, J. (1996). A patient care team approach to multicultural patient care issues. *Journal of Nursing Care Quality, 10*(3), 75–79.

Phillips, L. R., & others. (1996). Toward a cross-cultural perspective of family caregiving. *Western Journal of Nursing Research, 18*(3), 236–251.

Price, J. L., & Cordell, B. (1994, August). Cultural diversity and patient teaching. *Journal of Continuing Education in Nursing, 25*(4), 163–166.

Putsch, R. W. (1985). Cross-cultural communication: The special case of interpreters in healthcare. *Journal of the American Medical Association, 254,* 3344–3348.

Sanjur, D. (1995). *Hispanic foodways, nutrition and health.* Needham, MA: Allen & Bacon.

Sluzki, C. C. (1984). The patient-provider-translator triad: A note for providers. *Family Systems Medicine, 2,* 397–400.

Spector, R. E. (1996). *Cultural diversity in health & illness* (4th ed.). Stamford, CT: Appleton & Lange.

Spicer, J. G., & Others. (1994). Supporting ethnic and cultural diversity in nursing staff. *Nursing Management, 25*(l), 38–40.

University of Washington, Healthlinks. (1996). *http://healthlinks.washington. edu/clinical/ethnomed/eritrean.html*

Waitzkin, H. (1984). Doctor-patient communication. *Journal of the American Medical Association, 252,* 2441–2446.

Washington, H. (1997, October 26). Fear of medical care can become deadly. *EMERGE.*

Watchtower Bible and Tract Society. (1992). *Family care and medical management for Jehovah's Witnesses.* New York: Watchtower.

Waters, C. M. (1996). Professional development in nursing research—A culturally diverse postdoctoral experience. *Image: Journal of Nursing Scholarship, 28*(l), 47–50.

West, E. A. (1993, September/October). The cultural bridge model. *Nursing Outlook, 41,* 229–234.

Williamson, E., Stecchi, J. M., Allen, B. B., & Coppens, N. M. (1997, January/February). The development of culturally appropriate health education materials. *Journal of Nursing Staff Development,* pp. 19–23.

Yoder Wise, P. S. (1995). Cultural diversity in healthcare. In S. Yoder Wise (Ed.), *Leading and managing in nursing.* St. Louis, MO: Mosby.

Websites: *www.tcns.org, www.diversityrx.org, www.geocities.com,* and *www.interaccess.com*

Consulates and Embassies

Consulate General of **Argentina**
12 West 56th Street
New York, NY 10019
(212) 603-0400

Embassy of **Belize**
2535 Massachusetts Avenue, NW
Washington, DC 20008
(202) 332-9636

Consulate General of **Bolivia**
211 East 43rd Street
New York, NY 10017
(212) 687-0530

Consulate General of **Brazil**
630 5th Avenue, Suite 2720
New York, NY 10111
(212) 757-3080

Embassy of **Cambodia**
4500 16th Street, NW
Washington, DC 20011
(202) 726-7741

Consulate General of **Cape Verde**
607 Boylston Street, 1st Floor
Boston, MA 02116
(617) 353-0014

Embassy of **China**
2133 Wisconsin Avenue, NW
Washington, DC 20007
(202) 625-3360

Consulate General of **Colombia**
535 Boylston Street, 11th Floor
Boston, MA 02116
(617) 536-6222

Consulate General of **Costa Rica**
80 Wall Street, Suite 718
New York, NY 10005
(212) 425-2620

Consulate General of
Dominican Republic
20 Park Place, Suite 1124
Boston, MA 02116
(617) 482-8121

Consulate General of **Ecuador**
800 2nd Avenue
New York, NY 10015
(212) 808-0170

Consulate General of **El Salvador**
46 Park Avenue
New York, NY 10016
(212) 889-3608

Embassy of **Eritrea**
910 17th Street, NW
Washington, DC 20006
(202) 429-1991

Embassy of **Ethiopia**
2134 Kalorama Road, NW
Washington, DC 20008
(202) 234-2281

Embassy of **Greece**
2221 Massachusetts Avenue, NW
Washington, DC 20008
(202) 667-3168

Consulate General of **Guatemala**
57 Park Avenue
New York, NY 10016
(212) 686-3837

Embassy of **Haiti**
2311 Massachusetts Avenue, NW
Washington, DC 20008–2802
(202) 332-4090

Consulate General of **Honduras**
486 Beacon Street, Suite 2
Boston, MA 02115
(617) 247-2007

Embassy of **India**
2107 Massachusetts Avenue, NW
Washington, DC 20008
(202) 939-7000

Embassy of **Japan**
2520 Massachusetts Avenue, NW
Washington, DC 20008
(202) 238-6700

Embassy of **Laos**
2222 S Street, NW
Washington, DC 20008
(202) 332-6416

Consulate General of **Nicaragua**
61 Broadway, Suite 2529
New York, NY 10006
(212) 983-1981

Embassy of **Nigeria**
1333 16th Street, NW
Washington, DC 20036
(202) 986-8400

Consulate General of **Panama**
1212 Avenue of the Americas
New York, NY 10036
(212) 840-2450

Consulate General of **Paraguay**
1 World Trade Center
New York, NY 10048
(212) 432-0733

Consulate General of **Peru**
535 Boylston Street, 3rd Floor
Boston, MA 02116
(617) 267-4050

Consulate General of **Portugal**
899 Boylston Street, 2nd Floor
Boston, MA 02116
(617) 536-8740

Puerto Rican Economic
Development Administration
666 Fifth Avenue
New York, NY 10103–1599
(212) 245-1200

Embassy of **Russia**
2650 Wisconsin Avenue, NW
Washington, DC 20007
(202) 298-5700

Embassy of **Saudi Arabia**
601 New Hampshire Avenue,
NW
Washington, DC 20037
(202) 342-3800

Embassy of **Somalia**
600 New Hampshire Avenue,
NW, Suite 710
Washington, DC 20008
(202) 342-1575

Embassy of **Vietnam**
1233 20th Street, NW, Suite 501
Washington, DC 20036
(202) 861-0737

Index